STOP YOUR INDIGESTION

CAUSES • REMEDIES • RECIPES

by Phyllis Avery

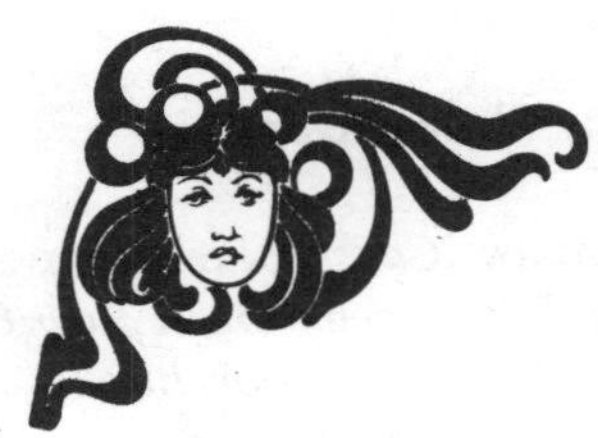

HYGEIA PUBLISHING COMPANY
1358 Fern Place
Vista, CA 92083

Although the authors and publisher have exhaustively researched all sources to ensure the accuracy and completeness of the information contained in this book, we assume no responsibility for errors, inaccuracies, or omissions. Readers should use their own judgment and consult a holistic medical expert or their personal physician for specific applications to their individual problems.

ISBN 1-880598-36-1

Avery, Phyllis, 1936-
Stop Your Indigestion: Causes, Remedies, Recipes

Other books by Phyllis Avery:

Stop Your Tinnitus: Causes, Preventatives, and Treatments
The Garden of Eden Recipe Book Raw Fruit & Vegetable Recipes
The 10-Minute Vegetarian Cook Book

HYGEIA PUBLISHING COMPANY
1358 Fern Place
Vista, CA 92083

Graphics by Alonna L. Farrar, A. Boyd-Farrar Graphics, Vista, California

Typeset by SuperScript Word Processing, La Mesa, California

Printed in the United States of America

TABLE OF CONTENTS

Part II: Remedies for Indigestion

PART III: RECIPES

ACKNOWLEDGEMENTS

For their professional help in contributing to this book, I wish to express my deep appreciation to the following people:

Dr. T.C. Fry
Dr. Herbert M. Shelton
Dennis Nelson
Victoria BidWell
Marti Wheeler
William F. Welles, D.C.
Ralph C. Cinque, D.C.
Dr. Vivian V. Vetrano, D.C., M.D.
Mike Benton
Otto Carque
Ken Pelletier, Ph.D
Dr. Alan Immerman
Hannah Allen
Dr. William Esser
Stanley S. Bass, D.C.
Susan Hazard, Ph.D.
Dr. John M. Tilden

Special thanks to T.C. Fry for editing this book and to my typesetter, Evelyn Vincow, for the many improvements she made.

FOREWORD

Why Americans Are Unhealthy

Two powerful superstitions are impeding the welfare and progress of the human race. The one is the conviction that disease is an entity, a mysterious something that attacks us from the outside without warning, either in the form of germs or as inclemency of weather. The other -- perhaps the more harmful of the two -- is the belief that for each disease specific remedies, such as drugs, serums, vaccines, etc., must be found, and that when we are afflicted, we have to submit to a specialist's treatment or even to the removal of the affected parts or organs.

The misconceptions have prevailed so long because of that characteristic trait in the average individual which always leads him to try to shift the responsibility for his sins of omission or commission to some outside cause rather than to hold himself to account for the violation of nature's laws, and because of the almost universal ignorance of the fact that disease is merely an effort on the part of nature or the universal life force to restore normal conditions in the organism.

Our present system of commercialism has taken advantage of this situation by misleading people through clever advertising to persist in their errors in order to maintain the demand for drugs and serums, proprietary medicines, and artificial foods and drinks. These entail not only an enormous pecuniary (monetary) loss, but also an appalling impairment of health.

Otto Carque, author of
the classic book *Rational Diet*

ABOUT NATURAL HYGIENE

The concepts and recipes in this book are based on the teachings of natural hygiene. Natural hygiene bases itself upon meeting the needs of humans, strictly in accordance with their biological disposition.

Some important concepts of natural hygiene are as follows:

Health is normal and natural to humans just as with all creatures in nature. Health is produced only by healthful practices.

Disease, sickness, ailments, and suffering are abnormal, unnatural, and unnecessary. Unhealthful practices inevitably produce disease.

All healing is self-healing. Nothing in the world outside of the body's faculties has the power and intelligence to assess body problems and to create the cells and fluids necessary to effect tissue repair. "Treatments" from the outside can never substitute for the biological processes and always instead interfere with them. Diseases do not have to be prevented. They will not happen unless caused.

Health can be regained and maintained only by healthful living. All that is introduced into or onto the body other than those life essentials normal and natural to the body is harmful.

INTRODUCTION

I am not a medical doctor. All the knowledge I have regarding indigestion has been learned mainly from books, lectures, health retreats, and the experiences of my family and friends. What's more, any subject you wish to learn is available because all knowledge has been recorded. Medical libraries across the country are accessible to all.

This book offers insight as to how indigestion occurs, other information to stop your indigestion, and recipes for avoiding indigestion. The more understanding we have about indigestion, the more we can visualize what is happening in our bodies, and with that comes the motivation to change our dietary habits.

In spite of the fact that there have been dozens of authoritative books available over the years addressing the problem of indigestion, about 98% of Americans continue to suffer from digestive disorders. I have read every book available on the market, and, with few exceptions, most of the recommendations did not help my family. What we are being told in the many books, pamphlets, and articles on the market is evidently not working. Worse yet, although every orthodox medical book admits ignorance of what causes the problems related to indigestion, the medical industry prescribes "cures" for diseases it doesn't fully understand.

The purpose of this book is to demonstrate to you how this needless suffering can be eliminated from the American scene. It aims to help sufferers of indigestion understand the very basics of how the body functions, thereby protecting against the medical/pharmaceutical complex, which is trying to convince the public that indigestion is a normal occurrence and that taking a multitude of nostrums is the natural way to solve the condition.

Most importantly, good health is our birthright. Illness is an unnatural condition. Most of us were born healthy.

When illness strikes, it is usually caused by our disobedience of the laws of nature.

Note: indigestion is a catchall having no precise medical meaning. Nausea, heartburn, flatulence, belching, abdominal pain, and vomiting all have been called indigestion.

Disclaimer: we should never try to diagnose our own afflictions. When symptoms such as severe or persistent pain, nausea, abdominal swelling, vomiting (especially any which brings up blood), diarrhea, constipation, and dizziness occur, one should get a diagnosis from a doctor.

We spend the first half of our lives wasting our health to gain wealth, and the second half of our lives spending our wealth to regain our health.

-- Author Unknown

PART I
CAUSES OF INDIGESTION

INDIGESTION

Americans entertain themselves via the mouth. They eat for taste sensations rather than for the purpose of nourishment. Consequently, over 50% of the meals in this country result in indigestion and some degree of intestinal distress. Rumblings in the stomach are indications of digestive problems. Smelly gas emissions are symptomatic of poor digestion. Heartburn, belching, nausea, foul breath, and coated tongue are also manifestations of poor digestion.

That over 100 *billion* doses of antacids and "digestive aids" a year are reportedly taken to alleviate the discomforts of the human food tube is further evidence of the great prevalence of indigestion. According to the *Wall Street Journal*, the number-one-selling prescription drug in the United States is an antacid for stomach disorders -- Tagamet. In spite of the long list of poisonous effects of this drug listed in the *Physician's Desk Reference*, medical doctors continue to prescribe it.

It's interesting to note that we are the only species in the world that, when finished eating, medicates itself to ease the suffering of indiscriminate eating.

Antacids work by chemically neutralizing excess hydrochloric acid in the stomach brought on by poor eating habits. Most antacids contain aluminum compounds*, which are especially risky for people with kidney problems.

---

*Antacids that contain aluminum include these brands: Rolaids, Amfogel, Camalox, Digel, Gelusil, Maalox, Mylanta, Riopan Plus, Tums, Titralac, and Someco. There may be others, and formulas change; always check labels.

The level of aluminum salts in your blood doubles when you take such antacids. Heavy use may affect your body metabolism and your ability to process certain essential minerals, and may lead to bone abnormalities. More and more evidence reported from the scientific community names aluminum as one of the causes of Alzheimer's disease.

Bicarbonate compounds also widely used as antacids include sodium bicarbonate (baking soda) and potassium bicarbonate. Sodium-ion bicarbonate increases the sodium level in the body and may be risky for those with high blood pressure.

Unfortunately, most people don't know that celery, bok choy, broccoli, lettuce, and other highly alkaline vegetables are better antacids than most antacid potions and pills. For instance, each rib of celery is equal to several pills in acid-neutralizing power. What's more, celery is a usable food that also furnishes the needed nutrients and bulk to dilute the seething mess and cause its dispatch from the stomach. As an antacid, freshly-made celery juice is more effective than eating whole celery.

The widespread overuse of laxatives is understandable, since over 90% of Americans suffer constipation constantly or sporadically. Prolonged use of laxatives seriously injures peristaltic nerves and muscles, thus causing even further impairment.

Remedies for diarrhea are also abused. One of the most popular antidiarrheal drugs, diphenoxylate hydrochloride, is a narcotic substance that can cause addictive symptoms; an overdose can be fatal. To prevent overdose, the drug is formulated with other substances that can cause dry skin, flushed face, rapid heartbeat, and other dangerous side effects.

Acid stomach can lead to ulceration and even cancer if its assaults are continued over the years. Antacids aggravate the condition even though they neutralize the acids.

When acid stomach arises, the body uses its ready reserves of alkalis. When these are exhausted, it robs its bones of calcium, magnesium, iron, etc, in order to neutralize the acids. This results in osteoporosis of the bones and teeth. In teeth this shows up eventually as cavities. The teeth are usually sabotaged from within rather than from without.

Heartburn occurs when food in the stomach backflows through the esophageal sphincter into the esophagus. **It's strange that no one questions why what came down the tube so comfortably earlier should be so burning after an interval in the stomach.**

Meat-eaters should take note of the fact that about 6% of meat is usually uric acid. We have no uricase or other enzymes to break down alien uric acid, hence the body must deal with it as a non-metabolizable acid and get it out of the system. This is done by neutralization, the combining of the uric acid with the body's own base salts, especially the calcium of the bones. Unfortunately, much of this neutralized uric acid ends up in joints, causing what is called arthritis. There is a long list of other diseases in which acid indigestion is implicated.

The nourishment our body receives is determined by the food we digest and assimilate. Food not digested is passed through the alimentary canal. In fact, the digestive tract uses more energy than any other organ of the body. Actual damage occurs when undigested food becomes soil for bacteria. The resulting putrefaction and fermentation by-products, when absorbed, irritate and poison our cells and tissues.

Repeated cycles of indigestion or poor digestion deny us needed nourishment. Toxic substances frequently absorbed contribute to headaches, backaches, colds, the flu, pneumonia, asthma, arthritis, sinusitis, acne, cancer, allergy, constipation (by disabling peristaltic nerves and muscles), and a long list of other pathologies.

Diseases of the stomach, intestines (diverticulitis), colon (colitis), and rectum are on the increase. In general, the medical establishment treats these diseases with drugs and surgery, but such treatment does not remove their *underlying causes*. If we wish to remedy this situation, we must adopt a sane plan of living that includes sound nutritional principles.

The archaic notion that we need to eat from each of the four basic food groups at every meal is probably responsible for more digestive difficulties than any other dietary habit we have. Man is the only animal in nature that combines, on average, fifteen different foods at one sitting. Animals in the wild eat only one food per meal.

There are no long-term advantages to eating the conventional American diet. Haphazard and indiscriminate eating may offer immediate gratification, but in the long run, the ultimate result is disease and early death.

Much of the information in this book was supplied by T.C. Fry, Dean of the American Health Sciences Institute and Director of Health Excellence Systems. He suffered from acid indigestion for many years and kept antacid pills within hand's reach at all times. Since everyone around him suffered from the same obvious symptoms of indigestion, he considered the problem a "normal" occurrence. On Thanksgiving Day in 1970, he started to read a book that had lain dormant in his library for sixteen years. It was Dr. Herbert Shelton's *Superior Nutrition*. He finished the book at one sitting and passed up Thanksgiving dinner. That very day, Fry changed his dietary habits; his indigestion ceased, never to return again.

DIGESTION OF FOODS

Most of the food substances taken in by the body for nourishment require some alteration before they can be absorbed into the blood and in this way carried to all parts of the body. The conversion of foodstuffs into assimilable substances is known as digestion. For example, proteins are broken down into amino acids, carbohydrates are converted into simple sugars, and fats are broken down into fatty acids. The body absorbs and uses these simple substances for the constant building of new tissues.

Dennis Nelson explains in his book, *Food Combining Simplified**, that the human digestive tract may be divided into three cavities -- the mouth, the stomach, and the small intestine. Each of these cavities contains its own distinct digestive secretions with which to carry on its own specific work of digestion. In each of these three stages, the work carried on at one stage prepares the food for the digestive work done at the next stage.

When food enters the mouth, the mechanical process of mastication (chewing), along with the chemical process of insalivation (mixing with saliva), initiates the digestive process. The taste buds are excited, and these tiny nerve endings send signals to the brain to determine the type of food ingested. Immediately, specific juices are secreted, and an environment is created for the efficient digestion of that particular food. If this food contains starch, then a specific enzyme called *salivary amylase* (ptyalin) will also be secreted in the saliva.

Swallowed food passes down the esophagus and into the stomach, where the digestive process continues. Here we find gastric juice containing primarily hydrochloric acid and digestive juices. The acidity of this gastric juice ranges from highly acidic to mildly acidic or nearly neutral,

---

*See Recommended Reading.

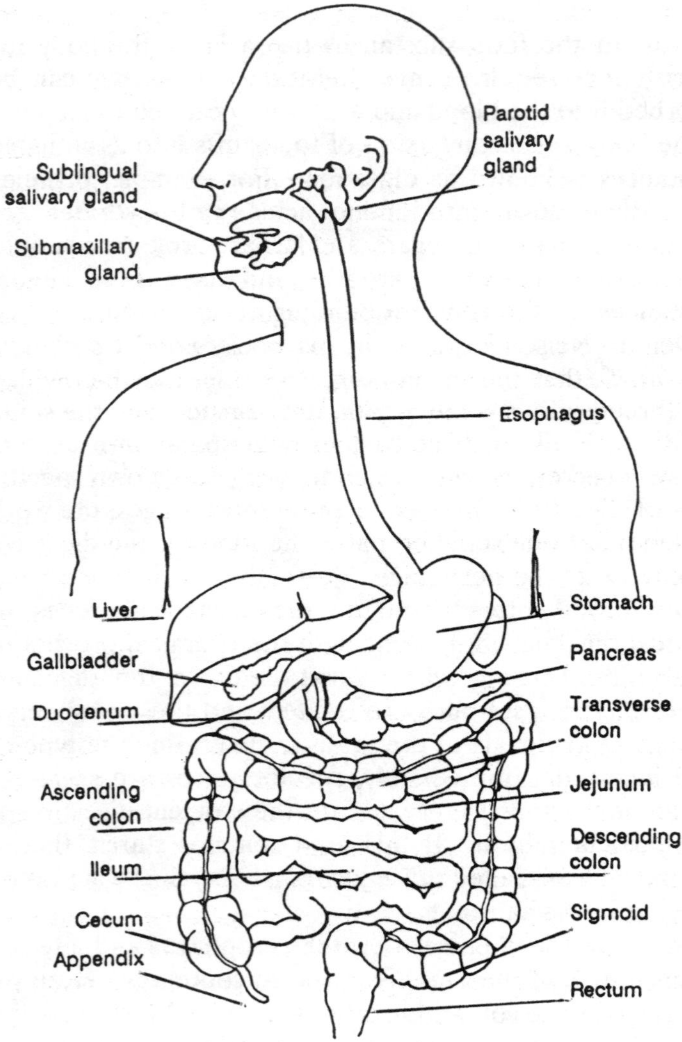

Figure 1. Diagram of the gastrointestinal tract from the mouth to the rectum.

depending on the type of food eaten.

Also present in the gastric juice are three primary enzymes: *pepsin*, which acts upon proteins; *gastric lipase*, which acts upon fats; and, in a minority of people, *rennin*, which acts upon milk proteins.

The important fact to understand here is that each enzyme can act only upon one class of food. For instance, the enzyme salivary amylase, which acts upon starches, cannot act upon protein or fat. In fact, enzymatic action is so specific that each one of the different forms of complex sugars, such as maltose or lactose, requires its own specific enzyme for its digestion.

An additional consideration is the fluid medium in which the digestive process takes place during the gastric phase. In the case of starches, salivary amylase requires an alkaline medium in which to continue its work and will be destroyed by a highly acid environment. The enzyme gastric lipase and its action upon fat are also inhibited by a highly acidic medium in the stomach. However, in the case of proteins, we have an opposite situation. They require a highly acid environment for the enzymatic activity of pepsin to take place. This is created by a sufficient outpouring of hydrochloric acid into the gastric juice.

As previously stated, the three stages of digestion require the action of different enzymes, and the efficiency of their work is determined by the digestive efficiency of the preceding stage. For example, if pepsin, the enzyme secreted in the stomach during protein digestion, has not converted these proteins into *peptones*, then *erepsin*, the enzyme secreted in the intestine, will not be able to carry on the final stage of protein digestion -- that of converting the peptone into amino acids. The work of each enzyme is designed *specifically* for that stage at which it is secreted.

Nelson concludes that in order for a food to be efficiently digested, the limitations of each stage of the digestive process must be respected. This requires that a food be eaten by itself or in combination with other foods that will not interfere with the distinct activity of different enzymes. When two foods are eaten that require opposite conditions for their digestion, the secretions poured out will interfere with each other and digestion of both foods will be limited or even suspended.

CAUSES OF INDIGESTION

1. Eating foods together that are incompatible in digestive chemistry.

2. Eating "foods" that humans are not biologically equipped to digest easily and efficiently.

3. Eating foods with different digestive times.

4. Eating foods that contain condiments, preservatives, seasonings, irritants, imitation flavorings, heated oils, etc.

5. Eating fermented foods.

6. Eating predominantly cooked foods.

7. Eating beyond digestive capacity, or overeating.

8. Eating when emotionally upset or physically or mentally fatigued.

9. Drinking liquids with meals.

10. Gulping down food.

11. Eating frequent meals.

12. Eating too close to bedtime.

13. Eating when ill.

14. Lack of vigorous exercise.

15. Taking certain pharmaceutical and other drugs.

16. Smoking cigarettes.

1. Incompatible Food Combinations

Man is the only animal that must have as many as 30 different foods at one sitting.

-- Dr. John Brosious, 1969

If we do not eat proper foods properly combined, our stomachs become battlegrounds!

-- Dr. Herbert M. Shelton

In an article written by Arden Conard, N.D., D.C., for *Healthful Living* magazine (August 1985, p. 56), Conard explains that proper food combining is basic to health. It is simply based on our natural biological heritage, including fundamentals of structure and physiology. Nature's way demands simplicity, and our desire to alter this plan will be met with less than ideal consequences. To combine foods properly is to eat only foods of compatible digestive character at one meal. It does not refer to attempting to get all the essential amino acids in certain amounts at each meal. This effort is unnecessary because it has been discovered that the body does indeed store amino acids from meal to meal and day to day to draw upon as needed -- in fact, about four pounds of them as labile protein.

There are only three major categories of foods: proteins, carbohydrates, and sugars.

Protein requires an acid medium for digestive breakdown into amino acids, which are the building blocks for tissue repair, enzymes, etc. Proteins are such foods as nuts, seeds, beans, meat, milk, and other dairy products. It is with protein foods that the greatest care must be exercised in food combining, because the putrefactive by-products of undigested protein are highly toxic.

Starches require an alkaline digestive medium. The alkaline medium facilitates the breakdown of carbohydrates into simple sugars like glucose and fructose, which are the only forms of carbohydrate the body can use. Incompatible food combinations cause fermentation, which produces toxic by-products, primarily alcohol. Starches are such foods as potatoes, carrots, corn, dry beans (also high in protein), grains, yams, and winter squashes.

Fruits require an alkaline digestive state. When ripe, they are predigested. This is the true food of humans. Fruits are ideal foods as developed for us in nature. Fruits are pure -- they contain no toxic substances, as vegetables often do. Fruits contain amino acids, simple sugars, fatty acids, vitamins, and minerals. They furnish every human dietary requirement. Fruits are subclassified into three categories: sweet, subacid, and acid.

T.C. Fry states that when protein foods (which require an acid environment in the stomach for their digestion) and starchy foods (which require an alkaline stomach environment for their digestion) are eaten together, indigestion usually results. The stomach, of course, cannot be acid and alkaline at the same time. Chemically, alkalis and acids are opposites; they neutralize each other.

When incompatible foods are eaten, they are retained by the stomach. They ferment, in the case of undigested starches and sugars (as in fruits and starches), or they putrefy or rot, as in the case of undigested proteins and amino acids. The reason for this is simply that they stay in the stomach too long. It is warm and moist in the stomach. Bacteria will proliferate and do what nature intended them to do -- break down unused organic matter. Fermentation causes alcohol to be produced in the digestive tract, with the same consequences as imbibing and with the same potential for liver damage.

The digestive glands react to the foods eaten to the best of their ability. They interpret the signals they receive and

Food Combining Chart for Complete and Efficient Digestion

Proteins
(Concentrated Foods)

Bean sprouts
Coconut
Dairy products*
Dried beans
Dried peas
Garbanzo sprouts
Lentil sprouts
Meat/fish/poultry*
Nuts (raw)
Nut butters
Seeds
Seed butters
Soybeans
Sunflower sprouts

*Not recommended, but included for clarity.

POOR

POOR — **Oils** / **Fats** / **Avocados** — **GOOD**

Starches
(Concentrated Foods)

Artichokes
Beets
Carrots
Chestnuts
Coconuts
Grains
Jerusalem artichokes
Lentils
Limas
Mature corn
Parsnips
Pasta
Peas, mature
Potatoes
Pumpkins
Rutabagas
Split peas
Turnips
Winter squash
Yams

GOOD **GOOD** **GOOD**

Non-Starchy Vegetables (High Water Content Foods)

Asparagus
Broccoli
Brussels sprouts
Cabbage
Celery
Chard
Collards
Corn (new)
Cucumber
Eggplant
Endive
Escarole
Green beans
Kale
Kohlrabi
Lettuce
Okra
Parsley
Spinach
Sprouts
Summer squashes
Sweet pepper
Tomatoes*
Watercress
Zucchini

*Tomatoes don't combine well with starches.

Acid Fruit		Low-Acid Fruit		Sweet Fruit	Melons
Blackberries	Plums (sour)	Apple	Kiwi	Bananas	Cantaloupe
Grapefruit	Pomegranate	Apricot	Loquat	Cherimoya	Casaba
Kumquat	Raspberries	Blueberries	Mango	Dates	Crenshaw
Lemon	Strawberries	Cherries	Nectarine	Dried fruit	Honeydew
Lime	Tangerines	Figs (fresh)	Papaya	Grapes (Muscat	Musk
Orange	Tangelos	Grapes	Peach	and Thompson)	Persian
Pineapple		Huckleberries	Pear	Persimmon	Sharlyn
		Plums (sweet)		Raisins	Watermelon

- Melons are best eaten as a separate meal from other fruits.
- Eat fruit by itself on an empty stomach, unmixed with other foods except lettuce and/or celery.
- Let 1-2 hours elapse after eating fruit before eating other foods. Wait 3-5 hours after a protein meal before eating fruit.
- Avocados are best combined with low-starchy vegetables. They make a "fair" combination with starches or acid fruits.
- Eat only one protein food at a meal.
- Fats inhibit the digestion of protein.
- Never drink liquids with or immediately following a meal.

supply the best secretions they can muster to preserve the health of the organism. When a saturation point is reached, due to continuous bombardment from intolerable food combinations, the ability of the overworked digestive system to make the necessary adaptations is reduced or destroyed, and disease is the result.

Thus, the more foodstuffs you eat, even if they are foods to which we are biologically adapted, the more likely that you'll ingest foods that present chemical conflicts and even chemical affinities that render them partly or wholly indigestible. Such unusable foods become poisons that devitalize and inflict suffering upon the system.

While I was working on the manuscript for this book, a new book was published about Elvis Presley's diet. The title is *The Life and Cuisine of Elvis Presley*. The author, David Adler, tells about Elvis's craving for peanut butter and banana sandwiches fried in margarine. Less than a year before Elvis died, he flew from Memphis to Denver in his private plane to feast on fool's gold loaf, a gargantuan peanut butter and jelly sandwich in a hollowed loaf of Italian bread, topped off with a pound of fried bacon.

It is probable that the constant turmoil in Elvis's body was a contributing factor in his taking so many drugs. Now that you know from my book what detrimental effects poor eating habits have on the body, can there be any doubt that Elvis is dead?

The following combinations of foods are the *least* compatible with the human digestive system. Although these combinations are commonly eaten because the eater experiences no immediate adverse reaction, the cumulative adverse effects will surface later on in life. We should take heed of Dr. Herbert M. Shelton's statement:

"YOU CAN'T VIOLATE A SINGLE PRINCIPLE OF NATURE AND FAIL TO SUFFER FOR IT! YOU'LL SUFFER FOR IT WHETHER YOU REALIZE IT OR NOT. YOUR BODY DOES

NOT ALWAYS MAKE YOU CONSCIOUSLY AWARE OF THE PROBLEMS YOUR BAD HABITS IMPOSE UPON IT!"

Acid/Starch Combination

All acids destroy salivary amylase, the starch-splitting enzyme in the saliva, and thus arrest starch digestion in the mouth and stomach. Additionally, because of the different digestive times of fruits and starches, the fruits will be detained in the stomach awaiting digestion of the starch. This leads to fermentation of the fruit sugars.

Bad Examples:

Pizza (tomato and wheat)
Yams with pineapple or other fruits
Tomato-based soup with potatoes or rice
Orange juice and cereal
Spaghetti and tomato sauce
Potato salad using lemon or vinegar

Protein/Starch Combination

Proteins require an acid environment, and starch requires an alkaline environment for digestion in the stomach. It is not possible for two processes to occur at the same time. The highly acidic medium will destroy the salivary amylase.

There is an exception to this rule when eating raw, mildly starchy vegetables. Carrots, cauliflower, zucchini, and other such vegetables can be eaten with nuts and seeds.

Bad Examples:

Meat and potatoes
Pumpkin pie with cream topping

Peanut butter (all butters) and bread
Mashed potatoes (milk and butter)
Eggs and bread
Meat sandwiches
Chili (meat and beans)
Fish and rice
Chicken and noodles
Ham and beans
Cereal and milk
Macaroni and cheese
Potatoes and eggs
Potato chips and sour cream dip

Protein/Protein Combination

Not only are proteins the most difficult to digest, but gastric acidity, type, strength, and timing of secretions for various proteins are not uniform. Eating two concentrated foods simultaneously may cause the food to rot, and rotten food not only cannot be assimilated but toxifies the body as well.

(Note: as I mentioned earlier, the most recent data concerning protein needs has shown that it is unnecessary to consume all essential amino acids at each meal.)

Bad Examples:

Turkey with nut stuffings
Omelets
Trail mix

Acid/Protein Combination

The enzyme pepsin will be active only in the presence of one particular acid: hydrochloric acid. Other acids may actually destroy pepsin, which is necessary for protein digestion.

There is an exception to this rule. Proteins such as nuts, seeds, and cheese decompose more slowly than other proteins because of their high fat content. The inhibiting effect of fat on the gastric digestion of protein causes these types of proteins to receive their strongest digestive juice during the latter part of digestion. Therefore, fruit acids do not delay the secretion of gastric juice any more than the fat content of these particular proteins already does. This distinction makes it acceptable to eat acid fruits with nuts or cheese.

Bad Examples:

Strawberry milkshake
Grilled cheese and tomato sandwich
Cranberry and turkey
Ham with glazed fruit
Yogurt with fruit

Fat/Protein Combination

Fat has an inhibiting influence on digestive secretions and lessens the amount and activity of pepsin and hydrochloric acid necessary for the digestion of protein. Because our need for fat is very small, and most protein foods already contain a sufficient quantity of fat, any additional fat intake makes digestion more difficult.

Bad Examples:

Avocado with sunflower sprouts or nuts
Scrambled eggs with butter
All fried foods

Sugar/Protein Combination

Sugars also inhibit the secretion of gastric juice, thus interfering with protein digestion. This is true of fruit sugars, white refined sugar, maple syrup, and honey.

Bad Examples:

Snacks with nuts and honey
Ham and brown sugar

Sugar/Starch Combination

If starch is combined with sugar, the starch is disguised, preventing the adaptation of the saliva to starch digestion. This combination produces indigestion and therefore prevents the body from assimilating food.

Bad Examples:

Fruit-filled pastry
Pies and cakes
Juice and/or fruits with cereals or breads
Yams and brown sugar
Snacks with coconuts and honey
Doughnuts

The true cause of impaired health lies in our failure to comply with the laws and requirements of life. All health problems arise from the abuse of natural laws, not from the correct use of them.

-- Harvey Diamond

2. Foods Humans Are Not Biologically Adapted to Eat

Forbear, mortals, to pollute your bodies with the flesh of animals. There is corn; there are the apples that bear down the branches by their weight; and there are the grapes, nuts, and vegetables. These shall be our food.

-- Pythagoras, 582 B.C.

We are the living graves of murdered beasts, slaughtered to satisfy our appetites.

-- George Bernard Shaw, 1940

Flesh Foods/Red Meat, Fish, Fowl, Legumes, and Most Grains

Humans' structure and digestive systems show that we evolved for thousands of years living on fruits, nuts, seeds, and vegetables. The diet of any animal corresponds to its physiological structure. During the last Ice Age, humans resorted to eating animal flesh in order to survive. The custom of eating meat continued after the Ice Age, either by necessity, through habit, conditioning, or through lack of realization of the damage it caused.

Man is not a carnivore and does not secrete uricase, the enzyme needed to break down uric acid for its elimination. The stomachs of carnivorous animals have ten times as much hydrochloric acid as noncarnivorous animals and thus can digest fibrous tissues and bones. The digestive tract of a carnivore is only three times the length of its body. Since flesh decays very rapidly, the products of this decay quickly poison the bloodstream if they remain too long in the body. A short digestive tract permits rapid expulsion of putrefactive bacteria and decomposing flesh.

MEAT EATER	LEAF/GRASS EATER	FRUIT EATER	HUMAN BEING
has claws	no claws	no claws	no claws
no pores on skin; perspires through tongue to cool body	perspires through millions of pores on skin	perspires through millions of pores on skin	perspires through millions of pores on skin
sharp, pointed front teeth to tear flesh	no sharp, pointed front teeth	no sharp, pointed front teeth	no sharp, pointed front teeth
slightly developed incisor teeth	no upper incisors	well-developed incisor teeth	well-developed incisor teeth
no flat molar teeth to grind food	flat back molar teeth to grind food	flat back molar teeth to grind food	flat back molar teeth to grind food
rasping tongue	smooth tongue	smooth tongue	smooth tongue
small salivary glands (not needed to predigest grains and fruits)	well-developed salivary glands, needed to predigest grains and fruits	well-developed salivary glands, needed to predigest grains and fruits	well-developed salivary glands, needed to predigest grains and fruits

small salivary glands (not needed to predigest grains and fruits)	well-developed salivary glands, needed to predigest grains and fruits	well-developed salivary glands, needed to predigest grains and fruits	well-developed salivary glands, needed to predigest grains and fruits
acid saliva; no enzyme ptyalin to predigest grains	alkaline saliva; much ptyalin to predigest grains	alkaline saliva; much ptyalin to predigest grains	alkaline saliva; much ptyalin to predigest grains
much strong hydrochloric acid in stomach to digest tough animal muscle, bone, etc.	stomach acid 20 times less strong than meat-eaters	stomach acid 20 times less strong than meat-eaters	stomach acid 20 times less strong than meat-eaters
teats on abdomen	teats on abdomen	mammary glands on chest	mammary glands on chest
intestinal tract only 3 times body length so rapidly decaying meat can pass out of body quickly	intestinal tract 10 times body length; leaves and grains don't decay as quickly, so can pass more slowly through the body	intestinal tract 12 times body length; fruits don't decay as quickly, so can pass more slowly through the body	intestinal tract 12 times body length

Nature did not intend for man to eat flesh foods. Man's digestive tract is 12 times the length of his body. Meat passes very slowly through the human digestive system, taking up to three days. Vegetarian foods take only 16 to 30 hours. During this time, the disease-causing products of decaying meat are in constant contact with the digestive organs. The body's 30 feet of intestinal tract is forced to cope with decomposing food and its train of toxic substances. The habit of eating animal flesh in its characteristic state of decomposition creates a poisonous state in the colon and deranges the intestinal tract relatively quickly.

Short-term evidence of this poisoning includes constipation, heartburn, bad breath, mucus, foul stool, and offensive underarm odors. These symptoms may also be accompanied by such behaviors as irritability, impatience, nervousness, fatigue, insomnia, and depression.

Meats are promoted as being the best protein source available. Humans have so little hydrochloric acid compared with carnivores that we can't manage meat, especially when eaten with digestively incompatible starches, sugars, and acids. When cooked, the proteins of the meat coagulate and deaminate, and thus become inaccessible to human digestive juices. Again, bacteria putrefy (rot) the meat and produce a profusion of putrefactive by-products, resulting in indigestion.

Animal products contain virtually no fiber. Consequently, meat moves very sluggishly through the human digestive tract, making chronic constipation and hemorrhoids common ailments in our society. The American dinner invariably combines animal foods with starches (potatoes, beans, bread), which results in indigestion.

Animal products are not essential to the human diet. There is no vitamin, mineral, amino acid, or fatty acid that cannot be satisfactorily provided by a fruit and vegetable diet.

Foods of our biological adaptation will satisfy hunger, digest easily, and supply energy, clear-headedness, and emotional fitness.

Think of the fierce energy concentration in an acorn! You bury it in the ground, and it explodes into a great oak! Bury a sheep and nothing happens but decay.

-- *George Bernard Shaw*

What's Wrong With Eating Fish?

1. Fish is excessively high in protein and has *zero fiber.*
2. All high-protein diets are linked to osteoporosis and loss of calcium from the bones. Eskimos suffer from rampant osteoporosis, worse than any other culture. They begin to lose their teeth in their twenties as a consequence of their fish-centered diet.
3. High-protein diets are strongly associated with kidney disease, reducing by half the ability of the kidneys to function. There is a direct correlation between animal protein consumption and kidney stones.
4. High-protein diets are correlated to several forms of cancer: lymphoma, kidney, and colon cancer. Protein promotes cancerous growth of all kinds.
5. Fish contains no fiber. Thus, eating it compounds all the various problems -- from constipation to colon cancer -- connected with the lack of fiber.
6. Fish is high in cholesterol -- twice the amount in pork or beef. Crab, shrimp, and lobster contain the highest amount of cholesterol.
7. Fish becomes contaminated from polluted waters.
8. Fish has a relatively high rate of spoilage.

It is my view that the vegetarian manner of living, by its purely physical effect on the human temperament, would most beneficially influence the lot of mankind.

-- Albert Einstein, 1940

Milk and Milk Products

Cow's milk is not suited for human consumption. Milk is that "perfect food" provided by nature for the young of each mammalian species of animal. The nutrient content is specific for the nutritional needs of the particular animal. For instance, the milk of the cow is suited to the specific needs of the growing calf. Likewise, human milk is suited to the specific needs of the human infant. The enzymes rennin and lactase are present in sufficient quantities only in the gastric juice of infants. At about the age of three, when the child has a full set of teeth, the enzyme rennin begins to diminish. This phenomenon indicates the time for weaning and feeding solid food. There is no physiological need for milk from this time forth.

Animal milk is indigestible for most adults. Over 75% of the world's population cannot digest milk from animals. People often experience immediate poisoning effects: indigestion, gas, biliousness, constipation, cramping, coated tongue, headache, diarrhea -- all symptoms of autointoxication.

There is an element in all milk known as casein. Animal milks have three hundred times more casein than human milk. Casein coagulates in the stomach and forms large, tough, dense, difficult-to-digest curds that the four-stomach digestive apparatus of the calf can digest. But inside the human system, it becomes a thick mass of goo, and a tremendous amount of stomach energy must be spent in dealing with it. This results in lethargy. Some of this gooey substance hardens and adheres to the intestinal lining. Also, to rid itself of the toxic by-products of milk, the body secretes a great deal of mucus to carry it from the body.

If you are unable to "wean" yourself from milk, at least take milk alone so that your body can concentrate its digestive powers on it. Milks have high protein and fat content and combine poorly with all other foods. Upon entering the stomach, milk forms curds, which coat the particles of other foods in the stomach. This insulating effect prevents the digestion of the other foods until after the milk gets through the system. And if you must eat yogurt, don't consume it with fruit.

Also, if you insist on drinking milk, drink raw milk. Unfortunately, only two states, California and Georgia, are allowed to sell raw milk. Pasteurization of milk diminishes the nutrient value and the vitamin content; separates, thus making unavailable calcium and other minerals; destroys enzymes; is more likely to be constipating; and is more likely to lead to decay in teeth. Infants don't develop on pasteurized milk.*

Soybean and nut milks are excellent substitutes, having practically the same analysis as cow's milk, and the danger of disease is removed. Nut milks are in the recipe portion of this book.

Beans and Peanuts

Beans and peanuts are concentrated foods that contain protein, starch, and fat. As pointed out earlier, proteins and starches require different digestive media: the first

---

*Read Dr. William Campbell Douglass's book, *The Milk of Human Kindness Is Not Pasteurized*, listed in the Bibliography.

requires an acid medium, the second an alkaline medium. The conflict will neutralize digestive enzymes, resulting in fermentation and putrefaction.

Refined Grains

Since Americans consume a tremendous amount of *refined* grains, I will be addressing here the use of refined grains, rather than whole grains. The human organism has great difficulty digesting refined grains because they are much starchier than the human physiology can digest. In the animal world, animals who eat grains are called graminivores. They have sufficient amounts of salivary amylases that split starch. Man has only a scant supply.

Refined grains are practically devoid of natural fiber and moisture, causing constipation in some people and diarrhea in others.

Refined grains are addicting and fattening. Because of the lack of nutrition in refined grains, the body still hungers for the lost nutrients. This leads to overeating on more of the same and, finally, to addiction.

Junk Food

"Junk food disease" is the latest gastrointestinal offender to arrive on the American scene. It develops into a form of marginal malnutrition. The eating of fast-food hamburgers, soft drinks, pastries, candy, potato chips, French fries, pretzels, etc. causes severe abdominal pains, mainly among adolescents. Most gases from carbonated drinks are belched or burped.

The Standard American Diet is a pathogenic arrangement that is responsible for a long list of diseases. This is evident when a mere change in diet enables SAD Sufferers to become free of their problems and lead healthful lives!

-- *T.C. Fry, 1989*

Gluten in Grains

J.I. Rodale of *Prevention* magazine states that there are so many conditions caused by eating wheat that they are difficult to enumerate -- obesity, cavities, indigestion, colitis, constipation, and two dozen more.

In the case of celiac disease (called celiac in children, steatorrhea or nontropical sprue in adults) the abdomen is protuberant; stools are bulky, loose, pale, and frothy, with a foul odor caused by faulty intestinal absorption of fat and undigested starch. This leads to bacterial decomposition and toxic by-products. Alternating diarrhea and constipation result.

Gluten is a complex protein found in wheat, barley, rye, and oats. In a sensitive individual, the presence of gluten can derange the absorptive surface of the intestines, resulting in a massive deficiency of vitamins B_1, B_3, B_{12}, folic acid, and zinc. The symptoms of intolerance vary from mild upset stomach to a more serious condition in which the digestive system can no longer digest and absorb any food.

Note: wheat germ and bran do not contain gluten.

Baking Soda

Extensive tests have shown that the residues left in bread by baking powders retard the digestion of protein. Baking soda destroys pepsin and retards gastric digestion.

Gelatin

Gelatin products are artificially flavored and colored and packed with sugar. I have researched over 100 clinical laboratory tests that show a variety of physical problems caused by the use of gelatin, kidney problems being the most relevant to the subject of indigestion. Excessive use of supplements in gelatin capsules can cause constipation.

3. Combining Foods of Different Digestive Times

Men dig their Graves with their own Teeth and die more by those fated Instruments than by the Weapons of their Enemies.

-- Thomas Moffett, 1600

Eating foods with different digestive times causes the fast-digesting foods to be held up, resulting in fermentation. Also, if a protein is eaten with a carbohydrate, such as meat with bread or potato, the different digestive juices in contact with each other will nullify the digestion of each so that indigestion occurs. The protein will putrefy and the carbohydrate will ferment. The result is gas and flatulence in the system, with little value derived from the foods.

That which is not digested only wastes the body's energy in passing through the alimentary canal. Worse than this, the undigested food becomes soil for bacteria to feed upon, resulting in putrefaction and fermentation, which irritate and poison our tissues.

Bacteria convert starches and sugars into vinegars and alcohols, thereby affecting nerve cells. A single bout with fermentative indigestion can be responsible for the loss of hundreds of thousands of brain and nerve cells. This accounts for the early afternoon mental and physical slump many people experience. Alcohol is produced in the digestive tract, with the same consequences as imbibing it and with the same potential for liver damage. By recognizing our human digestive abilities, we greatly enhance our health and well-being.

This is not to say that applying the principles of food combining will insure good digestion; there are other factors that reduce our digestive capabilities, as previously listed.

The breakfast eaten by the average person is a dietetic nightmare. One of the worst and all too common practices is eating acid fruits such as oranges and grapefruit and following these with cereal or toast. The resulting indigestion and troubles are likely to be blamed upon the most wholesome part of the meal -- the fruit.

The human digestive system struggles to do the best it can with the haphazard combinations with which it is supplied. When young, strong and healthy, the body can do a reasonably good job of digesting bad combinations even though the tax placed upon it is enervating, hence disease-producing. But in the weak, the sick, and those with impaired digestion, it is urgent that correct food combinations be eaten if satisfactory digestion is to be achieved. The healthy person can make occasional compromises; the sick person should never do so.

Fruit with Starch or Protein

The sugars in fruits need little digestion and pass quickly through the stomach to the intestines for absorption in perhaps fifteen or twenty minutes. This is true of both fruit sugars and commercial sugars. Proteins are the most complex of all food elements, and their assimilation and utilization are the most complicated. The average time for meat to pass through the entire gastrointestinal tract is between 50 and 72 hours. Consequently, when fruit is eaten with slower-digesting food such as proteins or starches, the mix will be held up in the stomach and result in fermentation, with unpleasant symptoms.

Bad Examples:

Pies and cakes
Fruit and cereal
Nuts and honey bars
Meat or starchy vegetables cooked with honey or fruit

Protein with Starch

Although it's best to eat starches and proteins at separate meals, you can combine mildly starchy vegetables (carrots, cauliflower, zucchini, etc.) with nuts or seeds if all are raw.

Bad Examples:

Any flesh or dairy foods with potatoes, rice, beans, bread, or pasta

Fats with Proteins or Starch

Use fats sparingly. Fats delay digestion and thus the passage of starch from the stomach into the intestine. Fat not only inhibits the secretion of gastric juice, it also inhibits the physical actions of the stomach. Too much fat taken with a meal results in belching and a burning sensation in the throat.

When fats (avocados or nuts) are eaten with *raw* green vegetables, the inhibiting effect of fats on gastric secretion is counteracted, and digestion proceeds quite normally. The use of fat (avocados) with starch is considered acceptable, provided a green salad is included in the meal.

Bad Examples:

Bacon and eggs
Green pea and ham soup
Pie crust with cream filling

4. Condiments and Irritating Foods

Behold! I have given you every herb yielding seed,
Which is upon the face of all the earth, and every tree,
in which is the fruit of a tree yielding seed . . . To you,
it shall be for food.

-- *God* -- *In the Beginning*

Eating foods that contain condiments, preservatives, irritants (onions, alcohol, coffee, and chocolate), and toxic substances (vinegar) has an adverse effect on digestion. They irritate and impair the functional powers of the digestive organs and tract. Their harshness interferes with the signals to the glands that secrete digestive juices.

Condiments are addictive and increase one's appetite, creating artificial desire for a food that the body is not physiologically capable of digesting. Of course, this leads to indigestion.

Condiments are defined as substances that season and give relish to food. Examples are catsup, dressings, sauces, herbs, spices, relishes, mayonnaise, pickles, sugar, mustard, chili peppers, onions, garlic, vinegar, cayenne, horseradish, and ginger.

The highly poisonous essential oils in mustard, peppers, horseradish, cayenne, and other hot substances irritate the more delicate membranes of the digestive tract, increase peristalsis, and send the meal along the digestive tract without being digested, to be expelled in much less than normal time. Habitual use of condiments causes nature to thicken and harden the membranes from the mouth to the colon to protect against harm, and this lowers the vital tone of these organs.

The eating of condiments is an acquired, and thus unnatural, taste. Foods are no longer eaten for their own sake. Babies and toddlers find condiments repulsive. Condiments camouflage the fine, delicate flavors that nature puts into her food products and prevent the user from enjoying these finer flavors.

Condiments are toxic. The body reacts to the toxic inputs by diluting them so as to lessen the irritation. This results in chronic edema or water retention. The condiment user takes on a bloated appearance from head to toe, with swollen hands, legs, and feet, as well as puffy eyes and cheeks. Salt, the number one condiment in use, exhibits edematous qualities that contribute directly to toxicosis, high blood pressure, and weight gain.

Repeated irritation from condiments produces irreparable injury to the stomach, liver, intestine, kidneys, blood vessels, heart, and other vital organs. Catarrh, chronic inflammation, hardening of the arteries, glandular destruction, permanently impaired digestion, gastric ulcer, cancer of the alimentary canal, and colitis are among the results of using condiments.

Spices frequently cause an ulcerated colon, sometimes so severe as to require its surgical removal. Fortunately, at the onset of ulceration there is plenty of warning: cramps, pain, and finally bleeding.

Also, spices tend to inflame the intestines, causing increased blood flow and increased white blood cell production.

The only spices we use are made from organic, dehydrated vegetables. They are produced by the natural hygiene community. They are made from blending the powders of dried tomatoes, red peppers, parsley, sea vegetables, celery, and other vegetables. There are two sources for dehydrated vegetable seasonings.

Veggie Delight (on Catalog Sheet #2):
Ingredients: uncooked dried and ground tomato, onion, sweet corn, carrot, celery, beet, red bell pepper, spinach, parsley, sea vegetables of kelp or dulse, lemon solids, and selected herbs.

Veggie Volt (on Catalog Sheet #3):
Ingredients: uncooked dried and ground tomato, carrot, celery, red bell pepper, spinach, kelp, dill, parsley, yellow onion, lemon solids, and whole caraway and sesame seeds.

Monosodium Glutamate (MSG)

Monosodium glutamate is a flavor enhancer that causes gastric distress known as "Chinese restaurant syndrome." Symptoms, which often appear within 30 minutes after eating, include burning sensations in the neck and forearms, chest pain, and headaches. MSG is an indigestible non-food chemical.

Coffee and Tea

Coffee and tea inhibit the digestion of foods in the stomach, both because of the caffeine and other toxic substances they contain and because of the sugar that is commonly taken with them. Coffee is also a very strong stimulant of stomach acid.

Other items that contain caffeine are cola drinks, some cold remedies, medicines such as headache pills and No-Doz, and chocolate. All these forms are powerful stimulants of gastric juices that lead to heartburn and, eventually, ulcers.

Onions, Garlic, Etc.

All members of the onion family -- onions, garlic, leeks, shallots, chives, etc. -- as well as radishes and all other foods containing appreciable amounts of mustard oil -- inhibit digestion. All contain isothiocyanate, which causes irritation of the stomach and intestines just as it irritates the mouth and throat. Horseradish and mustard are especially strong in causing irritation, but ordinary white and red radishes also cause considerable irritation.

5. Fermented Food

Eating fermented foods such as vinegar, pickles, alcohol, sauerkraut, yogurt, kefir, some soy sauces, and so on, causes indigestion. All of these foods either retard or suspend digestion and therefore are not effective nutri-

tionally. Instead of adding nutritional benefits to the food, fermentation decreases some vitamin and mineral availability.

Fermented foods are a disaster in the diet. They perform no function, provide negligible nutrients, contain no "beneficial" bacteria, and have no magical life-extending properties. Additionally, fermented foods contain harmful bacterial waste by-products as well as preservatives, often salt, and vinegar.

Vinegar

Even a small portion of vinegar appreciably diminishes the digestion of starch. Vinegar contains acetic acid, which destroys ptyalin (salivary amylase). It also contains alcohol, which precipitates the pepsin of the gastric juice and retards or prevents gastric digestion of proteins. Processed pickles and salad dressings containing vinegar are unwholesome substances, an offense to the human digestive tract. Also, any fermented food, like apple cider or wine, will suspend all salivary digestion.

Alcohol

Alcohol inhibits the secretion of digestive juices, alters their chemistry, and destroys their enzymes, thereby suspending the process of digestion. Alcohol irritates the lining of the esophagus by direct chemical injury.

Folklore suggests that it is okay to drink alcohol with your meal because it stimulates the secretion of digestive enzymes. In actuality, alcohol is a local irritant and injures the stomach lining by causing erosion, swelling, and inflammation.

The American Digestive Disease Society states that alcohol causes more digestive problems, including the most serious forms of damage to the liver, pancreas, and stomach, than any other item in the average diet.

Refined food produces deficiencies.
Adulterated food produces toxicity.
Dead food produces death.

-- *Monte Kline*

6. Predominantly Cooked Foods

Homo sapiens is the only species on earth that eats cooked foods. All other animals eat their food in its natural state. With the exception of domesticated animals that are given cooked food to eat, man is the only species of the entire animal kingdom that suffers from a multitude of diseases.

Cooking is a relatively recent practice in the history of man. Obviously, very primitive man subsisted wholly on raw fruits, nuts, and green vegetables. Even when man started cooking animal flesh, it is probable that he still ate much of his other food raw.

According to Dr. Herbert Shelton, "Cooking destroys in part, if not wholly, the oxidizable factors of foods. This simply means that cooking 'burns' those portions of foods that the body ordinarily oxidizes. Once these substances have been oxidized, they cannot again be oxidized in the body; hence they are useless as food."

Cooking food destroys vital nutrients. Some vitamins are destroyed or lost. Some minerals are rendered unusable. Proteins are coagulated and deaminated, the amino acids are demineralized, and toxins are created in the alteration. Sugars are caramelized and disorganized. Fats are disorganized and rendered carcinogenic. Calcium becomes disassociated from organic compounds and thus becomes unusable to the body. Some unsaturated fats become saturated, then attach to and harden on the linings of artery walls. Starches are rendered less digestible. At 120° F and above, enzymes (the very life of the food) are totally destroyed.*

In cooking, natural fiber is broken down. Fiber is that part of the plant food which the body cannot break down enough to release its micronutrients. Uncooked, foods typically pass through the GI tract in 24 hours. When the same foods are cooked, however, the fiber is radically changed. It no longer occasions peristaltic action of the GI tract walls. An intestinal transit time of 48 to 72 hours is typical for cooked food. During this delayed transit time, the sugars are left to ferment, the proteins to putrefy, and the fats to turn rancid. These toxins are released and usually absorbed into the bloodstream. Autointoxication, therefore, takes place on a grand scale every time we dine on a cooked meal.

Cooked foods not only take longer to digest but often prove to be indigestible and inassimilable. Cooked foods quickly ferment and putrefy in the intestinal tract, causing digestive problems.

This is evidenced by the fact that the average conventional eater has about two pounds of intestinal bacteria, whereas eaters of living food have only a few ounces. About 20% of the feces of eaters of cooked food is dead bacteria, whereas eaters of living food excrete only a fraction of this as dead bacteria.

Enzymes are totally destroyed when the cooking temperature reaches 120° F. When the proteins of those

---

*The full explanation of this can be found in Victoria BidWell's book, *The Health Seekers' Yearbook*.

enzymes are destroyed, so are other proteins in the food. Likewise, other nutrients are deranged and destroyed. Over time, these nutrient deficiencies tax the body's ability to digest the debris of cooked food, which is toxic in itself. Further, cooked food is the underlying cause of disease.

All food in the raw state including enzymes contains living cells. If heat is applied to these cells, their proteins are coagulated, like the white of a cooked egg. If you cooked your food sufficiently to destroy each and every one of these live cells and tried to live on it, you would soon succumb to an array of degenerative diseases and die an early death. Fortunately, most persons eat fresh fruits and raw salads and food that is not cooked; hence, they can obtain sufficient nutrients to allow them to lead a sickly existence. Only raw food can totally and completely nourish the body and maintain it in good health.

Not only do raw foods contain all the nutrients necessary for good health, growth, maintenance, and repair, they do not poison the body and subject it to degenerative and debilitating diseases. Raw foods are rich in mineral content and are unfragmented by cooking. This means smaller quantities of food need be eaten to meet our needs. Fewer waste products result. Elimination is less. Improved endurance, greater strength, and clean fluid channels, together with excellent general health, both physical and mental, are a happy outcome.

A vast body of existing evidence shows that a predominantly raw diet can reverse bodily degeneration that accompanies long-term illness. Raw foods retard the rate at which you age and bring you seemingly boundless energy. You'll need less sleep. You'll even improve your emotional disposition. Raw foods provide more energy for the body, because much less energy is wasted eliminating the toxins resulting from cooked foods. All of these improvements are possible because raw fruits and vegetables are two to three times more efficiently utilized by the body than cooked foods.

In quite a short time, a predominantly raw diet does several things. The body's eliminative faculties more readily expel accumulated wastes and toxins. Optimal sodium/potassium and acid/alkaline balance are restored. Raw foods increase the microelectric potential of cells, improving the body's use of oxygen so that both muscles and brain are energized.

When most of your food is eaten raw, you'll eat less! A raw diet affords quick satiety on less food, hence does not overstimulate the digestive system and cause you to overeat. Raw foods are easily digested and expelled (16 to 24 hours, compared to 48 to 72 hours for cooked foods). Raw foods not only restore the natural appestat (appetite control), but they also help the body to achieve a normal weight. Obesity disappears quickly, safely, steadily, painlessly, and effortlessly.

Prolonged storage, freezing, drying, salting, and canning are all more or less destructive to the nutritional value of the food. Fresh vegetables stored at room temperature for only one day lose up to 50% of their vitamin C. Blanching and freezing destroy vitamins B_1 and B_2. Since up to 90% of the average American diet consists of cooked, frozen, or otherwise processed foods, it is no wonder that half of the population is suffering from various degrees of vitamin deficiencies and malnutrition, which develop into degenerative diseases.

What Happens to a Human Body That Eats Cooked Food

1. There is a rush of white blood cells toward the digestive tract, leaving the rest of the body less protected by the immune system. The immune system interprets cooked food as an invasion by toxins.

2. There is a general enlargement of white blood corpuscles in the blood and a change in the relative proportions of different blood cells. This phenomenon is called *digestive leukocytosis*.
3. The intestinal flora becomes putrefied, resulting in colonic dysfunction and allowing the absorption of toxins from the bowel. This phenomenon is variously called *dysbacteria*, *dysbiosis*, or *intestinal toxemia*.
4. Toxins and waste material build up in many parts of the body, including within individual cells. One of these toxins and wastes is called *lipofuscin*, which accumulates in the skin and nervous system, including the brain. It can be observed as "liver spots" or "age spots."
5. Malnutrition occurs at a cellular level. Because such a high proportion of cooked food consists of wastes and toxins, individual cells don't receive enough of the nutrients that they need.
6. The immune system, having to deal with the massive daily invasions of toxins, mutagens, and carcinogens, eventually becomes overwhelmed and weakened.
7. Autoimmune diseases occur (arthritis, rheumatism, multiple sclerosis, tooth decay, etc.). Parts of the body become so clogged with toxins and wastes that the immune system starts regarding them as foreign invaders that must be destroyed -- i.e., the body starts destroying itself.

7. Overeating

A drunkard may reach old age, but a glutton, never.

-- *Sylvester Graham*

Everything in excess is opposed by nature.

-- *Hippocrates*

This chapter draws heavily upon a lecture by Dr. Ralph Cinque and an article by Victoria BidWell.*

Obviously, overeaters suffer from indigestion. Even if one were to overeat a monomeal (a single-food meal), it would put a strain on the digestive system by putting more food in the body at one time than it can handle. Overeating is usually accompanied by burping, which is nature's message that you've had too much to eat.

Food eaten beyond digestive capacity is soil for bacterial fermentation, putrefaction and rancidity that ends up in a grand case of upset stomach. Food that spoils in your digestive tract supplies no nutrition; it only increases your level of toxemia. Average "unstretched" stomachs hold 3 to 6 cups of food, depending on the size of the individual. When you eat, there should be some room left in the stomach so that the food can mix and turn. Therefore, you should stop eating when 3 to 5 cups of food have been eaten, *before* your stomach is packed. If you have consistently overeaten, cut back by using the measurements as a guide, and your stomach will slowly shrink to normal.

---

*This material is compliments of Victoria BidWell and GetWell * StayWell, America! See Recommended Reading for details to receive GetWell's **free** 150-page catalog.

Eating beyond five cups of food is excessive. Certainly we all recall gluttonous holiday celebrations followed by unbuckling, moaning, groaning, and stupor. Usually a nap is necessary after such a tremendous meal, because the body has a limited amount of nerve energy, and nature places a priority on using that energy to digest the food.

A high-fat meal also lulls one into a trance-like state. The high fat content causes the red blood cells to agglutinate, that is, "stick together," and in that state, they carry less oxygen to the brain. "Food stupor" results.

Overeating causes emotional and mental problems. When one eats a heavy meal, his energy goes from his head to his stomach. All too often, physical sluggishness translates into mental sluggishness.

It has been estimated that the amount of energy expended to digest three conventional meals is the equivalent of eight hours of "working" energy. By selecting compatible food combinations, the digestive task is greatly lessened, thus allowing much more energy for discretionary use.

But how are we to know when we are hungry, and how are we to differentiate between genuine hunger and abnormal craving? One way to determine real from fictional hunger is where the hunger is felt. True hunger arises in the throat like thirst. The truly hungry person has no pangs, no gnawing feeling in his stomach; he is not weak, and he has no headache. If weakness follows a delay in eating, this is a sure sign of toxicosis. If the weakness is relieved by eating, this is further evidence of the stimulation that eating begets.

An individual with normal nutritional reserves in his body can omit a meal or more at any time without ill-feeling or loss of strength. Although true hunger is never manifested in the stomach but always in the mouth and throat, it is common to mistake distress in the stomach for hunger.

When overeating is the cause of stomach pain, a mild emetic to empty the stomach will often bring immediate relief. Warm two glasses of water, and add a half teaspoon of salt to each. Drink as much water as the stomach can hold. Put a finger down the throat after drinking the water, and the food will discharge out.

To lengthen thy life, lessen thy meals.

-- Ben Franklin

Overeating and Cooked Foods

Victoria BidWell stated that a major cause of overeating is the eating of cooked foods. Health is maintained only if the human body has the full range of nutrients needed and in the proper proportion. Not only are the essential nutrients destroyed by cooking, but cooking brings about changes in the nature of food proteins, fats, and fiber, rendering these food elements less usable. When the full range of nutrients needed is not available, the body is still "hungry" and crying for more food, regardless of the huge number of calories the diner may have consumed.

Because cooked food loses nutrients, color, and flavor, the food preparer overseasons the food to make it more tasty and stimulating. This promotes overeating because the food is so "irresistible" that the diner can't stop eating it. Addiction sets in. Loss of energy follows, and acute and chronic disease take the place of health and high energy.

It is important to note that eating very hot cooked foods damages the mucosal membranes of the mouth and esophagus as well as the lining of the stomach. The body has to expend even more energy to create new replacement cells for the irritated surfaces.

Note: see suggestions later in this section for practical ways to conquer overeating.

It is a requisite that men and women should be content with little and accustom ourselves to eat no more than is absolutely necessary to support life -- remember that all excess causes disease and leads to death.

-- Luigi Coronado, 1458-1560

8. Eating When Emotionally Upset or When Physically or Mentally Fatigued

When we use expressions such as "That makes me sick to my stomach" or "What's eating you?", or "I cannot swallow your behavior" or "I'm too depressed to eat," we are doing more than just using figures of speech. We are expressing, among other things, the role our feelings play in affecting our gastrointestinal tract.

Mental and emotional well-being is conditioned by many more influences and factors than merely physical well-being. While physical well-being arises from meeting the physical needs of the body correctly, this is not always enough to assure mental and emotional serenity. Repeated disturbances in function stemming from a person's emotional state can lead to actual diseases of the gut.

Dr. Herbert Shelton explains that good digestion depends upon emotional poise. Eating when digestive ability is low (as when one is emotionally upset, under tension or stress, feeling fatigued, or needing sleep and rest), eating soon after strenuous exercise, and eating during strong emotional experiences all hinder digestive processes by activating the sympathetic nervous system.

These conditions preempt blood and divert energy from the muscles to the skin and away from digestive faculties, thus inhibiting digestion. When one is relaxed, in contrast, the parasympathetic nervous system controlling digestion is fully functional and the digestive process is facilitated.

Proof of how emotions can disturb the organic function of the body is demonstrated when we blush under embarrassment, experience heart palpitations when excited, faint or involuntarily empty our bladder when fearful, cry when grieved, or tremble when angry.

The digestive system responds to mental suggestion or emotional unrest because the free manufacture and flow of all the secretions of the body depend on nerve energy, which is transmitted to all the organs of the body through an intricate network of nerves. Emotional stress or shock interferes with both the generation and transmission of nerve energy.

Under emotional stress, production of any or all of the digestive secretions -- saliva, gastric juice, pancreatic juice, intestinal juice, bile -- is suspended. Impairment of digestion will last during the entire period of shock or strong emotion until nervous balance is restored.

Dr. Shelton concludes that, because digestion bears the burden of emotional unrest, it is best to skip a meal if you are worried, apprehensive, grieved, angry, jealous, fearful, depressed, irritable, grouchy, etc. If hunger is unbearable, eat a very light meal, preferably of fruits. An undigested meal of flesh and starch will give rise to more poisoning than an undigested meal of fruit.

In many families, the dinner table is a battleground. All of the problems of the day are discussed, and arguments ensue. If this is your general pattern, the entire family's health would benefit by having family members eat at different times or in different locations in the home. Not only are you wasting money on food that will give no nourishment, you will add to your medical costs.

Ken Pelletier, Ph.D., states that the main ways to break the chronic stress patterns are stress management, diet, and exercise. Exercise breaks up both physical and mental tension. For example, the physiological effects of light exercise as a remedy for high blood pressure are comparable to, if not greater than, those brought about by drugs.

Pelletier concludes that any activity that you have in your life can be used like meditation. Prayer, walking, sex, play, running, singing, listening to Bach -- all allay stress.

See the suggestions later in this section for a stress-management program.

9. Drinking Liquids With Meals

Harvey and Marilyn Diamond have written in their best-selling book, *Fit for Life*, that without water our bodies would be reduced to a few pounds of minerals. Seventy percent of the body is water. Consider some of the functions of water in the body.

1. Water is necessary for assimilation in the body, from digestion and absorption to utilization and excretion.
2. Water delivers all essential food for life to all parts of the body.
3. Water collects wastes from all cells and transports them to the eliminative organs. Carbon dioxide, urea, and ammonia are some of the toxic substances that must be expelled from the body. Water carries them to the bowels, bladder, lungs, and skin for disposal.
4. Without sufficient water, we would have no saliva and wouldn't be able to swallow or talk. The gastric digestive juices in the stomach are practically all water.
5. Water provides lubrication and prevents excessive friction between tissue surfaces and joints.

6. Water, through evaporation on the skin, is the chief agent in regulating body temperature.

Given its important role, three considerations must be made. When should we drink water? What is the best kind to drink? How much should we drink?

Drink water when you are thirsty, except at mealtimes. Digestive juices exist in controlled amounts of body water, and drinking liquid, *any* liquid, with or after meals dilutes the digestive juice concentrations and passes them out of the stomach, thereby retarding digestion.

Following are guidelines of when to drink and when not to drink so as to enhance digestion:

Drink when thirsty, but wait 10 minutes before eating.

Wait 30 minutes after a fruit meal.

Wait two hours after a starch meal.

Wait three hours after a protein meal.

Morning, when the stomach is empty, is the best time to drink water. Tepid water is more acceptable than water that is hot, cold, or at room temperature.

If your thirst is unbearable during or after eating, eat celery stalks, lettuce, or cucumber spears, which are high in water content.

The best way to avoid excessive thirst during meals is to eliminate the use of salt and other condiments and to eat most of your foods raw or at most lightly steamed. Cooking deranges the nutrients in foods, and deranged nutrients are toxic, causing thirst. Since all fruits and vegetables are high in water content, they will provide you with all the water your body needs.

The best kind of water to drink, given today's contaminated environment, is distilled water, because it is the purest water available. *Water* is emphasized, not soda pop, which is a chemical concoction.

How much water should we drink? No amount can be specified, because the less water one gets from his food, the more one needs to drink. Other variables, such as body size, activity, and climate, must be considered.

Do not drink to some unscientific dictate such as "Drink eight glasses of water per day." We overwork our bodies if we consume water beyond the demands of thirst.

Humans are not naturally water-drinking animals. The only time you may experience thirst when you are eating properly is during periods of fasting, rigorous activity, or exposure to heat.

Drinking Alcohol

It is a myth that alcohol stimulates digestive enzymes. In actuality, alcohol harms the stomach's natural protective barrier -- a lining that prevents it from digesting itself. It inhibits the secretion of digestive juices, alters their chemistry, and destroys their enzymes, thereby suspending the process of digestion.

Some students drink deeply at the fountain of knowledge -- others only gargle.

-- Author Unknown

10. Gulping Food

Nature will castigate
Those who don't masticate.

-- *Upton Sinclair*

Eating too fast and not chewing food properly, especially foods like cereal grains that require thorough chewing and insalivation, will inevitably result in acid indigestion.

Poor mastication results in decreased saliva and enzyme flow. Gulped food is, therefore, poorly prepared for digestion. Because cooked food tends to be soft, it slips down the throat without need for mastication. Because eating is a chemical as well as a physical process, each stage must be properly executed. Mastication starts the digestive process along the entire alimentary canal, keeping the nerve communication channels open. If the food is poorly prepared for digestion, it follows that poor digestion will result in intoxicating fermentation and putrefaction products.

Even wholesome, well-balanced food will not be properly digested if eaten "on the run."

Chewing for Better Digestion

Digestion begins in the mouth. Chew your food thoroughly until it is liquid. Most important is the chewing of nuts and seeds until there are no solids left. Never use the moisture of foods like lettuce and tomatoes to help liquefy nuts or other concentrated foods -- chew them separately. The salivary glands will secrete sufficient moisture, and of the proper kind, for this purpose. Your foods will be better digested when you chew them thoroughly.

Natural hygienists suggest chewing your food between 35 and 45 times. Grains can take up to 75 "chomps" to pulverize and be thoroughly mixed with saliva. Nuts take even more chomps. For instance, for two almonds to be converted into a liquid cream would take about 125 chomps. But with thorough chewing, you will eat fewer almonds and get far more nutrition.

Physical, mental, and moral integrity constitute our most precious possessions -- a balanced, sound mind in a balanced, sound body. We have a moral obligation to ourselves, dear ones, society, posterity, and our Maker to strive for optimum health through obedience to natural laws governing health. The physical, mental, and moral health of the people of any nation is more important than its "gross national product."

-- Harry Kaplan, 1984

11. Eating Frequent Meals

Eat to live, and not live to eat. Many dishes, many diseases.

-- Ben Franklin

It's great to let food be a pleasure! Just don't let food be your only treasure!

-- Victoria BidWell

Dr. Vivian V. Vetrano*, former director of Dr. Shelton's Health School, addressed the subject of frequent meals as follows:

It is not possible to have good digestion when eating too frequently. If the small intestine is not ready to receive food, reflex action will cause a slower emptying time of the stomach, holding the present meal in the stomach longer than ordinarily, thus favoring bacterial decomposition, instead of normal digestion. Furthermore, when the stomach is filled before the previous meal has been completely digested in the small intestine, peristalsis increases in the intestines, hurrying along the previous meal to make way for the present meal. Consequently, the previous meal will not remain in the upper small intestine long enough for perfect digestion or absorption. When we eat all day long, much of the food is just passed through the intestinal tract undigested and unabsorbed. One who indulges in food too frequently is overworking the glands and muscles of the body simply for the palliation of symptoms or for the pleasure of the taste buds. This type of eating leads eventually and invariably to enervation, toxemia, disease, and premature death.

Digestion is muscular work. Partaking frequently of snacks keeps these muscles contracting so frequently that fatigue is inevitable. Future contractions are weaker, causing stagnation of food in the digestive tube, which may result in constipation.

Many people are afraid of not getting a sufficient supply of nutrients in the day so they constantly stuff themselves. Some have decided they have hypoglycemia because of having read an article on this popular new myth, and they place themselves on six meals a day because this is what they have read is good. Consequently, poor digestion is the rule instead of the exception.

---

*See information about Dr. Vetrano under Resources.

It is a cardinal sin to put food in a stomach that is not ready for it. It is the same as stoking a furnace when there is already enough fuel. You crowd both systems: in the furnace, complete combustion does not take place; and in the body, complete digestion is impossible.

Note: see Dr. Vivian Vetrano under "Resources" and "Recommended Reading."

Length of Time Between Meals

Efficiency of digestion concerns the emptying time of the stomach into the intestine. The three primary food groups each have a different transit time as they pass through the gastric pouch:

1. Fruits remain in the stomach an hour or less.
2. Starches require two to three hours to complete gastric digestion.
3. Proteins require approximately four hours.

Some more complex foods, such as dried beans, are rather difficult to digest. Due to their high concentrations of both starch and proteins, these foods may require five to six hours to complete gastric digestion.

The greatest tragedy that comes to man is the emotional depression, the dulling of the intellect and the loss of initiative that comes from nutritive failure.

-- Dr. James S. McLester
Former President, A.M.A.

Men do not die, they kill themselves.

Seneca, Roman philosopher

12. Eating Too Close to Bedtime

Eating too close to bedtime is another reliable cause of indigestion. Healthy digestion requires time coupled with mild activity.

Eating prior to a night's sleep can vary in time with the food eaten. If we eat easily digested monomeals of fruits not later than two hours before retiring, we should realize wonderful sleep. But if nuts, seeds, or heavy meals are eaten, bedtime should be delayed four or five hours.

Tell me what you eat and I'll tell you what you are.

-- Anthelme Brillat-Savarin (1825)

13. Eating When Ill

Whenever fever or inflammation is present, normal digestive energies are preempted by the body for crucial uses. Consequently, digestive powers are suspended almost completely. Since fruit requires a minimum of energy to digest and assimilate, fruit juice is the best food to consume should you elect to eat during illness.

Should a man, when ill, continue to eat the same amounts as when in health, he would surely die; while were he to eat more, he would surely die all the sooner. For his natural powers, already oppressed with sickness, would thereby be burdened with sickness, would thereby be burdened beyond endurance, having had forced upon them a quantity of food greater than they could support under the circumstances. A reduced quantity of food is, in my opinion, all that is required to sustain the individual into a long life.

-- *Luigi Coronado, 1458-1560*

14. Lack of Vigorous Exercise

If you don't find time for exercise now, you will have to find time for illness later!

-- *Wayne Pickering, 1982*

A strong body makes the mind strong.

-- *Thomas Jefferson*

Regular exercise is very important because a chronically inactive body atrophies and becomes sluggish, with greatly reduced body functions. If you suffer from chronic fatigue, poor sleep, digestive disorders, shortness of breath after little exertion, or poor posture, you are not exercising your body. You are directly and indirectly depriving your body of the energies that it needs to properly maintain its natural, healthful functions.

Regular exercise provides us with a stronger heart and lungs, increased metabolism, better digestion, good sound sleep, the elimination of a multitude of physical ailments, and especially with the energy to overcome stress.

(Victoria BidWell's book *The Health Seekers' Yearbook* covers this topic extensively with a step-by-step program based on your particular energy level. See Catalog Sheet #4.)

15. Taking Certain Pharmaceutical Drugs and Other Drugs

Medicine is only palliative. For back of disease lies the cause, and this cause no drug can reach.

-- Dr. Weir Mitchell

Any substance used in the body that contains chemicals is referred to as a drug for the purpose of this chapter.

Antacids

There are two kinds of antacids -- absorbable and nonabsorbable. Absorbable antacids like sodium bicarbonate disturb the acid-base balance of the blood and tissues, as well as the functioning of the kidneys, especially if given along with the ritual use of milk. Doctors no longer recommend absorbable antacids to their patients.

The aluminum compounds -- the hydroxide and the phosphate -- fall under the category of nonabsorbable antacids. They may cause constipation or diarrhea and are often combined with agents such as magnesium hydroxide to loosen the stool. Any aluminum in the body is an outright poison. Some scientists claim that excess aluminum might cause colon cancer.

Calcium carbonate, an ingredient in antacid that initially calms the stomach, in turn causes "acid rebound" by triggering the release of a hormone that stimulates the stomach to pump out *more* acid.

> *Man lives on one-fourth of what he eats. On the other three-fourths lives his doctor.*
>
> *-- Inscription on an Egyptian pyramid, 3800 B.C.*

Antibiotics

Antibiotics can cause nausea and vomiting.

Laxatives

Laxatives are destructive to health. They irritate the peristaltic nerves that set off the intestinal action called peristalsis. The constant usage of laxatives gradually destroys peristaltic nerves. Researchers have found that salt-based laxatives such as magnesium nitrate and milk of magnesia disrupt body chemistry or homeostasis. Oil-based laxatives prevent the absorption of needed vitamins and minerals; if continuously used, they can cause nutritional deficiencies.

Many physicians have encountered instances of ruptured appendix and peritonitis after a patient has taken a laxative for an attack of abdominal pain assumed to be due to constipation or indigestion but actually arising out of acute appendicitis. (Note: constipation is rarely associated with abdominal pain.)

Most physicians discourage anything more than an occasional use of glycerine suppositories as a laxative, because stronger remedies can cause severe irritation of the mucous membrane in the general area.

Aspirin

Aspirin eats away at the coating that protects the stomach from the acids that digest food. Studies show that aspirin causes one out of every seven hospitalizations for bleeding of the digestive tract.

Aspirin can cause gastritis (inflammation of the stomach lining). If aspirin use is heavy, it can cause gastrointestinal bleeding, aggravate ulcers, and bring on nausea and vomiting.

Codeine

Codeine is a narcotic which is derived from a poppy plant. It is used in the relief of pain and as a cough remedy. It is also used as an antidiarrheal drug, because it slows down muscle contractions in the intestinal wall. However, when taken over a long period of time, codeine may cause constipation and be addictive.

Tranquilizers

Tranquilizers may produce mild or severe symptoms of indigestion as a side effect.

Steroids

Large doses of steroids (cortisone) induce stomach and duodenal trouble. Although not directly related to indigestion, scientists reported that some patients developed lupus erythematosus (a degenerative disease of the connective tissues) and skin ulcers after receiving prednisone, a cortisone-like drug. Other reports show that cortisone interferes with the body's attempts to form collagen, the fibrous protein that is a necessary building block for bones, skin, and connective tissue.

Progesterone

Progesterone (a hormonal drug), causes heartburn.

Sorbitol

Sugarless mints contain sweeteners. The most commonly used sweeteners are xylitol, mannitol, and sorbitol, all members of the sugar-alcohol family. In sensitive people, they cause gas, cramps, and diarrhea. The reason for this is that they attract water when they're in the digestive tract. This can lead to diarrhea or other digestive upsets in some people. In addition, because they're not completely like other sugars, some may end up in the large intestine. When and if this happens, they become soil for the bacteria that live there, and more gas is created.

Products that contain sorbitol include medicinal syrups, gelatin capsules, foods, chewing gum, candies for diabetics and dieters, and certain toothpastes.

Opiates

Opiates can cause constipation.

What is impossible to see from the viewpoint of those who believe in "cures" is that the very symptoms the good doctors have suppressed and turned into chronic disease were the body's only means of correcting the problem! The so-called "disease" was the only "cure" possible.

-- Dr. Phillip Chapman, 1981

Four Rules about Taking Drugs

By taking drugs, we relinquish control of our health, explains Alan M. Immerman, D.C., in an article written for the *Truth Seeker* (Vol. 118, No. 1, 1991). The happy truth is that you can almost always feel better without using drugs and surgery. If you truly desire to take control of your health and become as full of vitality and vigor as possible, you must understand the basics of health philosophy.

Rule number one: *The foundation of health philosophy is that healing is a process accomplished by the body and only by the body.* External substances cannot exert curative actions on the body. Chemical drugs which are ingested are inert and lifeless and therefore cannot act. When such substances are taken, we are led to believe that the drug acted on the body, but this is impossible; *the body acts on them*. The body is the only source of healing.

When we swallow a foreign chemical, the body will either speed up or slow down the pace of normal activity. For example, examine the body's reaction to laxatives. The laxative is a powerful chemical irritant, so irritating that when it finds its way into the intestine, the body will feel so insulted that it will vigorously eliminate the irritant along with the intestinal contents. Would it be accurate to say that the laxative cured the constipation? No. The constipation developed because the intestine had been overworked and exhausted. The laxative did not make the intestine stronger or healthier in any way. In fact, since the chemical irritation of the laxative provoked the exhausted intestine to work very hard, the intestine will be weaker, not stronger.

Pneumonia and other infections may seem to be exceptions to the rule that drugs do not cure diseases. However, upon deeper analysis, we find that the rule holds true. Antibiotics will destroy the bacteria involved in the infection, but they will not cure the cause of infections, which is lowered body resistance. Only the body itself can work to increase health and resistance to the point where infections are rare.

Good health is a product of healthful living. Though healthful living itself cures nothing, it unleashes the body's healing power, which can do more than all the doctors in the world combined. Never underestimate this strength.

> *If anyone consults a doctor after the age of 30, he is a fool, since by that time everyone should know how to regulate his life properly.*
>
> *-- Tiberius, A.D. 30*

Rule number two: *The body almost always acts in its own best interests*. When you are acutely ill, many uncomfortable and distressing symptoms develop. These symptoms arise from the vigorous expression of the body's healing power. When the body eliminates waste material from the intestines or lungs, it is because the brain determined that health would be improved by such elimination. Attempting to suppress such symptoms with drugs makes one sicker, not healthier. There are rare exceptions, such as pneumonia, but this rule holds true 99% of the time.

The best doctors in the world are Doctor Diet, Doctor Quiet, and Doctor Merryman.

-- Jonathan Swift

Rule number three: *The short-term effect is opposite to the long-term effect.* A cup of coffee seems to increase energy, but, in fact, the long-term effect is more fatigue. Coffee gives the body no energy; it releases stored energy, thereby depleting the body further.

The flu is another example of the short-term effect being the opposite of the long-term effects. One feels terrible while the lungs and sinuses discharge waste materials. The short-term feeling is one of severe illness. Yet the long-term effect is better health. When the body harbors less of the waste material that has accumulated, the overall health level will be greater.

Rule number four: *Drugs and surgery should only be used as a last resort.* Drugs are powerful chemicals which have many negative side effects. Perhaps 100 changes in body function may follow using a drug, but of these, only 1 may be desirable and 99 undesirable. The 99 unwanted changes are called the side effects.

Drugs do not build health; they suppress symptoms at great cost. Turning off the fire alarm (the symptom) with a drug will not extinguish the fire (the cause of the symptom). Drugs can save lives in some cases, but most of the time they produce more harm than good.

Those who understand the basics of health philosophy can take control of their health.

16. Smoking Cigarettes

A short life is not given us, but we ourselves make it so.

-- Seneca, 62 A.D.

Cigarette smoking can induce chronic inflammation of the stomach -- chronic gastritis -- and clearly contributes to the symptoms of dyspepsia or indigestion itself. Smoking also increases the risk of developing ulcers, because it prevents the pancreas from secreting chemicals that neutralize stomach acids entering the duodenum.

Cigarette smoking is an irritant of the whole gastrointestinal tract. Smoking or sucking a cigar all day long can also lead to air swallowing, and thus to belching.

Of course, such intestinal problems are minor compared to the lung and respiratory tract problems that follow.

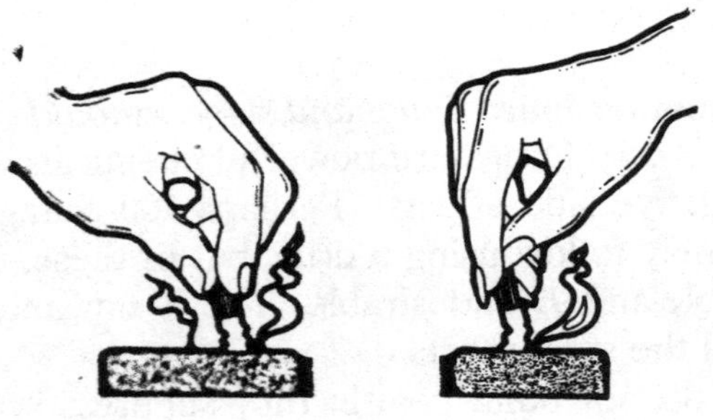

PART II
REMEDIES FOR INDIGESTION

SPECIFIC DIETARY REMEDIES

The information in this section is meant to help you make informed choices about your health. It is not intended as professional advice. It can serve to guide you through the confusing maze of modalities you may encounter. This section is a compilation of information from a dozen books written by physicians, Ph.D.'s, chiropractors, holistic physicians, and medical research writers; it also draws on discussions with pharmacists and from medical encyclopedias.

The following guide briefly describes problems of the entire alimentary tract and lists things you can do to relieve those conditions, should your lifestyle beget them. Of course, there is no substitute for healthful practices.

Note: the following symptoms warrant confiding in a health professional:

- Abdominal pain accompanied by tenderness
- Very serious pain, or pain lasting more than six hours
- Sudden change in bowel habits
- Vomiting blood
- Loss of weight or appetite
- Jaundice (yellowing of the skin and whites of the eyes)
- Fever lasting more than two days, or over 101 degrees

Colitis, Ulcerative Colitis, Crohn's Disease

Basically, these diseases are inflammations of the intestinal tract. Differences lie in location, severity, symptoms, and the extent of tissue affected.

Symptoms are a feeling of weakness through the abdomen, at times headache, often great pain and dizziness, emaciation, fever, weakness, and pains in various parts of the body.

Colitis is caused by a faulty diet. Constipation results from too many mixtures that irritate the stomach and bowels; too much of cane sugar products, grease, and white flour; eating too hastily; too much liquid and overcooked foods; taking cathartics; and food cooked in aluminum vessels.

Particular foods to avoid are milk and milk products, grains that contain gluten (wheat, oats, barley, and rye), chocolate, and caffeinated beverages. When drinking water, drink only distilled water.

A juice or water diet for a short time is advisable. When eating solid food, thoroughly chew and liquefy it with saliva, using no liquids with meals.

Suggested foods are papaya juice and raw cabbage juice. Avoid citrus juices, as they irritate the upper GI tract before their acids are metabolized.

Foods rich in zinc and vitamins A and C are beneficial because they are particularly needed by restorative faculties. Foods that are high in those nutrients are:

Carrots	Kale	Spinach	Turnip greens
Melon	Squash	Tomatoes	Persimmons
Apples	Yams	Broccoli	Sprouted grains
Guavas	Potatoes	Cabbage	Red bell peppers

Sunflower, pumpkin, or squash seeds

Avoid all roughage and foods containing skins and seeds until the condition clears up.

Surgery is of little use without changing your dietary habits. The surgeon can cut out the diseased portion of the bowel, but he can't stop the disease. In fact, studies show that 90% of those operated on for Crohn's disease have a second operation as little as two months later. And some doctors believe that surgery actually encourages the spread of Crohn's disease in the bowel.

Some doctors believe that drugs -- antibiotics, antihypertensives, anticoagulants, steroids -- can bring on an attack of colitis.

Constipation

The nature of the food eaten has much to do with normalcy or lack of bowel action. Chronic constipation is the accumulated effect of years of a faulty diet, such as eating the wrong foods, wrong combinations, hasty eating, poor mastication, low fiber, vitamin deficiencies, intestinal putrefaction, and fermentation. Emotional states and stress play havoc with normal bowel action. They usually lead to constipation but can sometimes cause diarrhea.

The prolonged use of laxatives and enemas actually worsens the constipation because it results in weak muscular tone and impairs muscular contractions of the colon. Different laxatives act in different ways. Mineral oil (and all oils that have been removed from their natural context, such as vegetable oils) coats the intestinal mucosa, thus preventing the absorption of nutrients. Oils also interfere with the digestion of carbohydrates and proteins. But oils eaten in their natural form, as in whole nuts, avocados, and seeds, are released slowly into the body. Since no coating develops to block either digestion or absorption, oil-bearing foods do not create constipation problems.

A better alternative to laxatives in severe cases would be the ingestion of psyllium husks. They absorb up to 60 times their weight in water to form a gel in the intestine, thus forming a bolus that must be moved out. Drink plenty of water upon rising and between meals. Also, flax seed soaked in distilled water two or three days is very effective in occasioning bowel movement. Drink only distilled water.

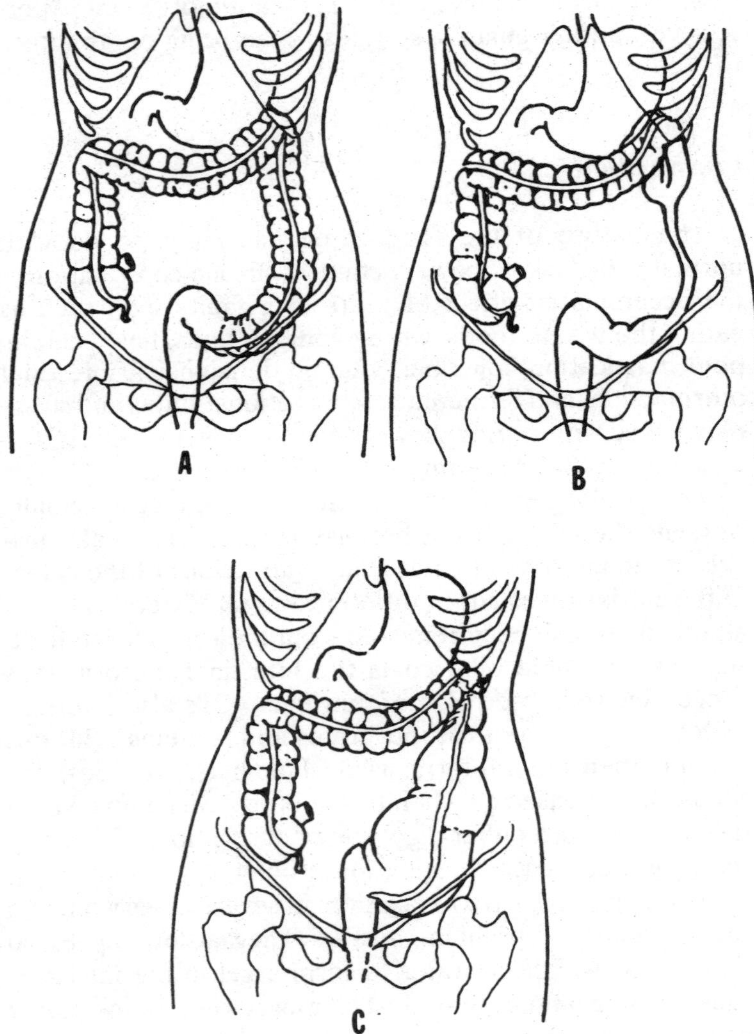

Figure 2. Diagram of normal and sick colons.

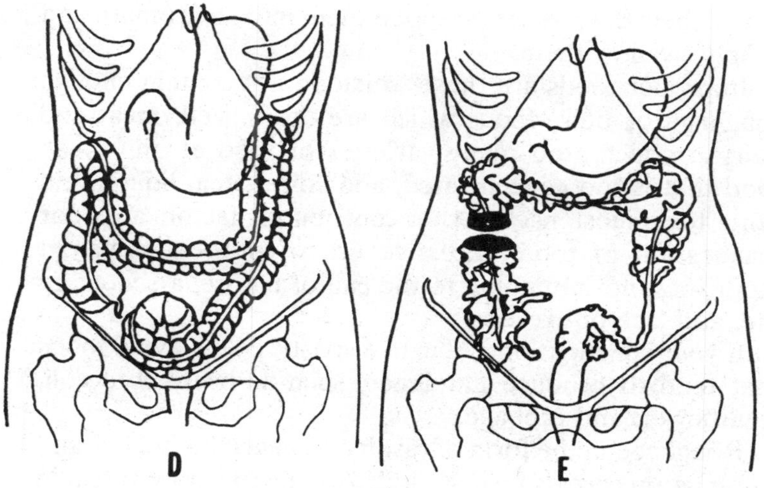

A, The normal large bowel or colon in the proper position in relation to other structures:

1, stomach; 2, appendix; 3, cecum; 4, ascending colon; 5, transverse colon; 6, descending colon; 7, sigmoid flexure; 8, rectum.

B, The colon in spastic constipation.

C, The colon in atonic constipation.

D, Ptosis (sagging) of the transverse colon, accompanied by displacement of the stomach.

E, Ascending colon, cut and opened to show small hole in the center of encrusted, hard fecal matter, probably more than 20 years of accumulation. The man whose x-ray is copied here thought his colon was healthy because he had daily movements.

Figure 2 continued.

Don't chew the flax seeds; spoon them into your mouth and simply swallow them.

Improper foods are those which do not contain enough roughage or bulk, foods which are devitalized, meat and dairy products, too many varieties of food at one meal, food that is too concentrated, and coffee, tea, liquor, and other toxic substances. Other contributing factors are poor mastication of food, excessive use of drugs and patent medicines, not attending to the call of nature, a sedentary life, and lack of exercise.

If your constipation is due to a spastic colon, avoid foods that tend to produce flatulence, such as beans, broccoli, cauliflower, and cabbage.

Roughage in the form of raw fruits, vegetable salads, and whole-grain cereals is suggested. Among the more valuable foods are dates and raisins (soaked), fresh figs (if dried, soak them), apples, bananas, cabbage (raw), carrots, beets, seeds, and nuts. Sprouted seeds are of great value.

Suggested juices are spinach, watercress, carrot, cucumber, celery, cabbage, beet, and tomato. These can be combined, but only according to proper food combining principles. Apple juice is also beneficial.

Avoid all refined and processed foods. Avoid salt, sugar, and white flour in any form. Avoid coffee, tea, and alcohol -- they interfere with peristalsis.

Drink one hour before meals or two or three hours after eating. Drinking with meals impairs digestion.

Exercise daily -- swimming, bicycling, gardening, tennis, horseback riding, brisk walking, or boating.

Use a small stool in front of the toilet to prop up your feet. (See Catalog Sheet #1 for a stool especially designed for this.)

In severe and persistent cases of constipation, my resources suggest a 10-day juice diet. The guidance of a natural hygienist is suggested. A list of natural hygienists can be found in the Resources section of this book.

Moderate exercise at least two hours after meals is advised. Never lie down or go to sleep just before or right after eating. Exercising at least an hour before eating oxygenizes the system, which in turn helps digestion. It is impossible to get the full benefit of your food without an exercise program.

Follow the squatting exercises at the end of this section.

A list of foods that tend to help you have regular bowel movements:

Prunes	Raisins	Turnips	Cabbage
Dates	Spinach	Squash	Brussels sprouts
Figs	Celery	Parsnips	Whole-grain bread
Apples	Lettuce	Carrots	Cauliflower
Pears	Corn	Pumpkin	Watermelon
Peaches	Okra	Walnuts	All citrus
Potatoes	Bananas	Cherries	Blueberries
Oat groats			

Foods that cause constipation:

Ryes	White bread	Cooked foods
Barley	Rolled oats	Hard-boiled egg
Meat	White rice	Browned-flour gruel
Cheese	Browned-flour gravy	

Note: The list of "constipating foods" above is for the purpose of clarity only. All of the foods listed should never be in your diet.

Diarrhea

Acute diarrhea is one of the body's best defense mechanisms. It's the body's way of hastening elimination of unwholesome substances from the system. This is why some doctors prefer not to prescribe antidiarrheal medication. Chronic diarrhea, however, can indicate a serious ailment (such as colitis) and should be checked by a physician. If they have no corrective measures, see a natural hygienist for courses you might follow.

Nevertheless, when you are suffering from this condition, you don't want to worsen it by continuing its causes. Below are suggestions to ease the discomfort and to help avoid future problems.

For parasitic diarrhea, avoid all foods for three days except applesauce made with raw, organic apples. After the condition improves, include millet and banana in the diet. Papaya is also recommended.

When you have diarrhea, it is suggested that you take only water until the body has purged itself. If you eat, take small meals, chewing food extremely well. Do not drink liquids with meals. I recommend a single food at a meal. Digestive capacity is low during diarrhea. Don't tax it with foods difficult to digest.

One of the major causes of diarrhea in this country is lactose intolerance. The cure, of course, is to eliminate milk and milk products from your diet. Only single foods like fruit juices and vegetables should be taken in simple, little meals until your intestines calm down.

All available fresh vegetable and fruit juices are beneficial for both acute and parasitic diarrhea.

Antacids are also a common cause of drug-related diarrhea. Maalox and Mylanta both contain magnesium hydroxide, so they act exactly like milk of magnesia. Antibiotics, quinidine, lactulose, and colchicine may also cause diarrhea.

Don't eat fatty, spicy foods, carbonated drinks, beer, beans, cabbage, cauliflower, Brussels sprouts, sweets, and salty foods. Avoid chewing gums; they contain sorbitol, which tends to have a laxative effect.

Replace potassium, which is depleted when you have diarrhea, by eating bananas and potatoes. You may ask your health care specialist about potassium supplements.

An ingredient that minimizes diarrhea is pectin. It is a fiber found in fruit, particularly apples, cherries, and bananas. Pectin allows water to be absorbed from the colon. Concentrated pectin can be found in health-food stores.

Also, get plenty of physical rest.

Diverticulosis

Before 1900, diverticulosis was a rare condition, but because of the advance in processed foods in America, more than half of Americans over 60 have diverticulosis. It is characterized by tiny, grapelike pouches or sacs (diverticula) along the outer wall of the colon. The average American gets about 16 grams of fiber daily, less than half of what he should be getting. But you should increase your fiber intake gradually over six to eight weeks to give your digestive system time to adjust.

In diverticular disease, numerous small pockets or sacs form along the wall of the colon or large intestine. These pockets form at weak spots in the bowel, where undue pressure and lack of tonicity cause the intestinal lining to bulge like a balloon. When one of the sacs becomes inflamed or infected, severe pain and cramping can occur.

Emphasis should be on high-residue foods such as raw vegetables and fruits, seeds, and nuts. Seeds and nuts should be ground up or chewed very well because particles can become lodged in the diverticula and, because of bacterial putrefaction, can cause inflammation. Sprouted seeds are excellent. If you eat cereals, suggested ones are millet, brown rice, buckwheat, and oat groats.

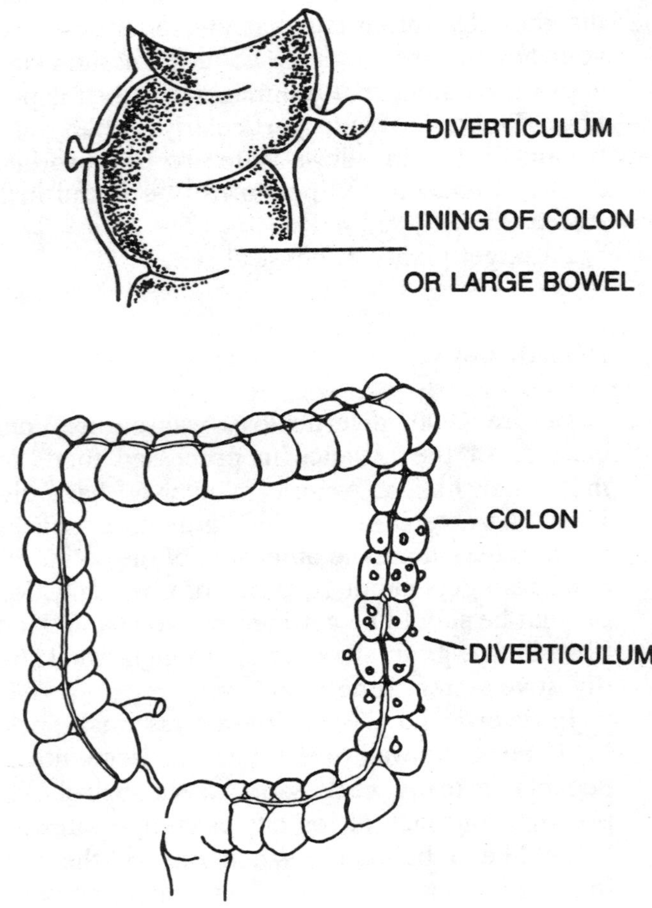

Figure 3. Illustration of diverticulosis.

Avoid all refined and processed foods, animal products, coffee, alcohol, chocolate, and tea -- they tend to irritate. Don't use suppositories -- they can become addicting. If a laxative is needed, eat soaked prunes along with the soaking water. Smoking also aggravates constipation.

The most practical and best source of fiber is pectin, found in apples, peaches, pears (leave skin on), cherries, bananas, pineapples, tomatoes, grapes, raspberries, avocados, raisins (soak them overnight in distilled water), and sunflower seeds.

If you can't get enough fiber in your diet, take psyllium husks. They can absorb up to 60 times their weight in water to form a gel in the intestine. Drink plenty of water upon rising and between meals. Psyllium husks are available in health food stores. Don't use bran, for the reason explained at the end of this section.

Squatting and situp exercises tone up the muscles in your colon. A slant board is also beneficial (see specifics after the section on squatting).

The quickest path to recovery from most problems is to fast as necessary for up to 3 weeks. See a natural hygienist for this (listed under Resources). A fast will enable your body to regenerate itself and restore some semblance of health and strength to the colon walls.

A deeper understanding of fasting would be helpful. Dr. Herbert M. Shelton's book *Fasting Can Save Your Life* is listed on Catalog Sheet #3. Paul Bragg's book *The Miracle of Fasting* is available in health-food stores.

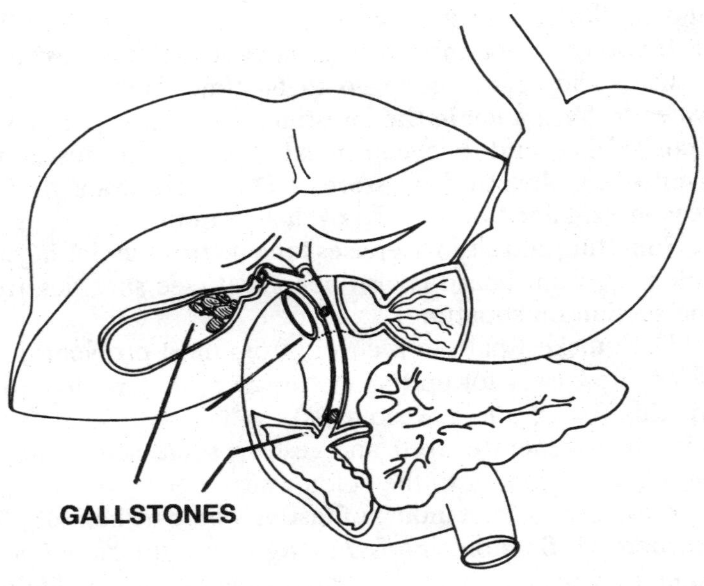

Figure 4. Liver, gallbladder, and pancreas.

The gallbladder sac lies under the liver. It stores some of the cholesterol/bile manufactured in the liver and assists in the process of digestion of fats in the stomach and the first part of the small intestine. Indiscreet eating over a period of years will cause the liver to overwork continually, producing a bile that is thick and loaded with excess waste. The more solid constituents of the bile, especially cholesterol and bile pigments, are precipitated, forming gallstones.

Gallstones may lie there quietly, but sometimes they migrate and temporarily get stuck in the narrow ducts leading from the gallbladder to the small intestine. When this occurs, you may feel faintness, nausea, chills, indigestion, or sharp, sudden, severe pains in the region of the liver (which is located under the right rib), extending to the right shoulder blade. There will be violent pains in the abdomen caused by the muscles becoming rigid, with tenderness manifested over the liver and general abdomen. The pain can be so intense that you vomit, become soaked with cold perspiration, and perhaps develop fever and chills. The attack may last a few minutes or a week. If you experience these symptoms, seek advice from a health specialist or physician.

Gallstones that lodge permanently in the bile duct will prevent bile produced by the liver from reaching your intestine. This, in turn, causes jaundice.

Over 92% of gallstones consist of inorganic calcium, as found in calcium tablets.

Because kidney stones are also composed of calcium and oxalate, physicians often recommend that people suffering from kidney stones reduce their calcium intake. Recent research, however, found that men who ate a diet rich in calcium had a 34% lower risk of developing kidney stones. It appears that oxalate is the real culprit, and adequate calcium can bind with dietary oxalate in the intestines, carrying it safely out of the body.

Excessive eating of refined grains, sugar, meats, eggs, fried and greasy foods, highly seasoned foods (especially salt), and dairy products are main causes of gallstones. If you have gallstones or kidney stones, restrict oxalate-rich foods such as beets (including tops), green peppers, spinach, Swiss chard, beans, blueberries, celery, chocolate, grapes, parsley, rhubarb, strawberries, summer squash, and tea. The use of hard water, bicarbonate of soda, any antacids with a calcium base, and too low a water intake are also causes. Generally, constipation and liver trouble occur before the gallstones form.

Keep your protein intake down. There is a direct correlation between the amount of protein eaten and the incidence of gallstones. Protein tends to increase the presence of calcium, uric acid, and phosphorus in the urine, which can lead to the formation of stones in some people.

Vitamin A is necessary to keep the lining of the urinary tract in shape and help discourage the formation of future stones. Natural foods are the best source. Eat plenty of carrots, apricots, broccoli, cantaloupes, pumpkins, and winter squash.

Activity is important. People who are sedentary tend to accumulate a lot of calcium in the bloodstream, and activity helps pull calcium back into the bones.

Doctors Robert R. Gross and Herbert M. Shelton, both natural hygienists, state that nothing clears the gallbladder like a fast. Fasting for even a few days (drinking only distilled water) will give immediate relief from the most intractable cases of gallstones. During the fast, the stones shrink gradually and eventually dissolve completely. Nothing clears out the liver as certainly as a fast. After a ten-day fast, supervised by a natural hygienist, go on a fruit diet, with emphasis on oranges, grapefruit, and unsweetened pineapple juice, for a week or ten days. Eat plenty of alkaline-forming foods (all vegetables except asparagus; all sprouts; all fruits except blueberries and olives; almonds and chestnuts; sunflower, sesame, and pumpkin seeds; green beans, peas, and snap beans).

Gross and Shelton say it is customary medical practice to dose the patient with pain relievers, but this is pernicious treatment and delays or suspends the passage of the stone or stones. A far less harmful mode of relief would be to put the patient in a tub of hot water. This should be done *gradually* so as not to shock the body. The water must be kept hot and should entirely cover the patient's torso. A cold cloth should be kept on his head. The patient should be kept in the hot water until the pain is relieved. If pain recurs when the patient is taken from the tub, this means that the stone has not passed, and he may be put back into the tub.

No food should be given so long as there is discomfort, nausea, or other signs of trouble. So long as there is nausea, no water should be given. Rest is imperative.

It should be known that there are no drugs which will remove gallstones, and also that olive oil is not effective in removing them.

Doctors Gross and Shelton conclude that surgery is necessary in rare instances in an emergency, but most surgery performed for gallstones is not necessary. Surgery does not remove the cause of stone formation; hence, it cannot remedy the real trouble. There is no shortcut to recovery, but practically all patients can get well if they will learn to live and eat properly.

Halitosis

The major causes of bad breath are caffeine, refined sugar, meats, beans, white flour, and cow's milk. These foods upset human biochemistry, resulting in the fermentation of carbohydrates and the putrefaction of proteins in the digestive tract. Noxious by-products enter the bloodstream and are passed out through the lungs.

Many cases of bad breath are caused by lung problems, gastrointestinal disorders, intestinal sluggishness, and particularly by chronic constipation. The unpleasant odor is usually caused by an exceptionally large amount of putrefied waste matter being absorbed into the blood and expelled through the lungs. In other words, bad digestion can mean bad breath.

The body is equipped to handle most gases generated internally without bloating, flatulence, or other discomforts. It is said that the average American has 7 to 10 quarts of gases created within the intestinal tract daily. Of this amount, only about half a quart is said to be "expelled." The rest is absorbed through the mucous membranes of the digestive tract and passed out through the lungs, often causing extremely bad breath.

Follow the recommendations under Causes of Indigestion.

Hemorrhoids

Hemorrhoids, or piles, as they are frequently called, are the most common GI tract illness.

Hemorrhoids are difficult to overcome, but three to four weeks of fasting and correct diet may largely overcome the condition. For those who don't have the luxury of going on a fast, follow the program for constipation, since it is considered a *major* cause of hemorrhoids.

A diet rich in fresh, raw fruits and vegetables and raw and sprouted seeds will improve circulation and the condition. Emphasis should be put on cabbage, red peppers, citrus fruits, black currants, seeds, and nuts. Totally eliminate from your diet all animal products, refined foods, and sugars.

Engage in a regular exercise program. Even walking is beneficial. Daily sitz baths will reduce the swelling and pain of hemorrhoids.

Sitz Baths

There are three kinds of sitz baths: hot, cold, and alternating hot-and-cold. The alternating hot-and-cold sitz bath has great therapeutic value for men's diseases, piles, constipation, dysentery, and diarrhea. Organs and glands of the pelvic region are stimulated and revitalized, and practically all body functions are beneficially affected.

For the alternate hot-and-cold sitz bath, two tubs are required. You can use large utility plastic tubs. One should contain water heated to 98-100° F; the other, water cooled to about 50-65° F. Enter either tub gradually. Extreme temperature changes shock the body. The water should cover the abdomen. Massage the hips and abdomen well. Keep a small blanket or heavy, large towel over the body above the water. Sit first in hot water for five minutes, then switch to cold water for five to ten seconds. Repeat twice. Do this two or three times a week.

Hernia

A hernia is the protrusion of an organ or part of an organ through a weak area in the muscle or cavity that normally contains it. The term is usually applied to a protrusion of the intestine through a weak area in the abdominal wall. In *hiatal hernia*, the stomach protrudes through the diaphragm into the chest.

The first symptom of a hernia is usually a bulge in the abdominal wall. It can be accompanied by abdominal discomfort. Problems that accompany hernias can be triggered by coughing, vomiting, sudden physical exertion, pregnancy, obesity, or the collection of fluid in the abdomen.

Chocolate, coffee, cola drinks, garlic, onions, peppermint, tobacco, aspirin, and certain drugs all worsen the condition by weakening the esophageal valve.

T.C. Fry of Health Excellence Systems states that the quickest correction is a period of fasting in order to detoxify and heal what is remediable. Then a raw food diet of mostly fruits with a regular program of fresh air, sunshine, and exercise will enable the body to strengthen its musculature and again create fitness -- both internal and external.

Fry concludes that hiatal hernia and many other types of hernias are resolved with a well-rounded program of exercises. However, many cases never respond completely or even at all. Nevertheless, an exercise regime has its benefits in all cases.

Other recommendations are as follows: lose weight if necessary, avoid bending or stooping, don't bend forward to scrub floors or weed the garden, don't wear tight belts or girdles, wait at least two and a half to three hours after a meal before lying down, sleep with your head elevated eight to ten inches, and avoid taking estrogen drugs, which aggravate heartburn.

Surgery is required in only about five percent of hiatal hernia patients, when there is a potential that the herniated stomach will pinch off the esophagus, bleed, or damage the lung or heart. Unwarranted hiatal hernia surgery can be expensive and risky and may produce new symptoms far worse than any associated with the original discomfort.

Pancreas

The pancreas serves as a source of both digestive enzymes and insulin. The digestive juices of the pancreas contain enzymes that break down proteins into amino acids, starch into sugar, and fat into a more soluble state. The pancreas also secretes insulin and glucagon into the bloodstream in relation to the level of glucose (blood sugar) in the body.

The symptoms of pancreatitis are weight loss, a decrease in the body's muscle mass, flatulence, and disturbance in the lower bowels and colon. Because pancreatitis will result in enzymic and vitamin deficiencies, other symptoms could be night blindness, inability of the blood to clot, abnormal bleeding, discoloration of the skin, bleeding from the GI tract, softening of the bones, bone pain, and bones that easily fracture.

The major causes of pancreatitis are denatured foods, combinations that form fermentation in the stomach, alcoholic drinks, and the use of cow's milk, which occasions the secretion of mucus as a carrier to take it through the mucous membranes. When the pancreas becomes inflamed or hardened, it does not secrete enough enzymic juices to digest properly the food in the intestines. Disease of the pancreas leads to other serious diseases such as diabetes.

The immediate treatment for pancreatitis is resting the pancreas by stopping all food.

Topical treatment consists of applying hot/moist heat to the spine, stomach, liver, and pancreatic area. Eat a diet of freshly made fruit juice for several days, followed by mainly raw fruits and fresh vegetable salads.

Tumors

There are many kinds of tumors. They are named according to the tissues involved, such as glandular, muscular, fibrous, and fatty. There are also cancerous tumors. Any of these tumors may enlarge rapidly and become ulcerated.

Tumors are invariably caused by impure blood and impurities of the system, unbalanced diet, constipation, and the inactivity of all the organs of elimination -- lungs, liver, kidneys, skin, and bowels -- therefore poisoning the system. The poisons accumulate around or in the weakest organs or where the body has the predilection to put them. Then the body encapsulates the toxins to quarantine them.

The first step in healing tumors is to cleanse the bloodstream by thoroughly relieving constipation and making all the organs of elimination active. For the first ten days (shorter or longer depending on the condition of the patient), drink orange, grapefruit, and pineapple juices only. Don't mix them. Drink at least six glasses of juice a day. After that, drink juices for five days. The ideal ones are celery, cucumber, parsley, lettuce, and carrot. These can be mixed. Eat a diet of oranges, grapefruit, apples, blueberries, red raspberries, cherries, peaches, pears, strawberries, avocados, pineapples, and tomatoes. All fruit should be well ripened to be fully beneficial.

Get plenty of fresh air and exercise, preferably in the sunshine, to cleanse the lungs and increase the circulation.

Ulcers

Dr. Robert Gross explains in an article published by Health Excellence Systems that pain consistently experienced in the upper abdominal region a few hours after eating is generally symptomatic of "typical" ulcer. Patients describe the pain as piercing, sharp, and burning. Coughing up of blood may be evidenced, as well as blood in the stool. Symptoms differ; other patients characterized the sensations as gnawing hunger. These sensations are extremely distressing. To offset the uncomfortable feeling, sufferers may eat large amounts of food, or they may continually consume food in lesser quantities, especially before going to bed.

Peptic Ulcers

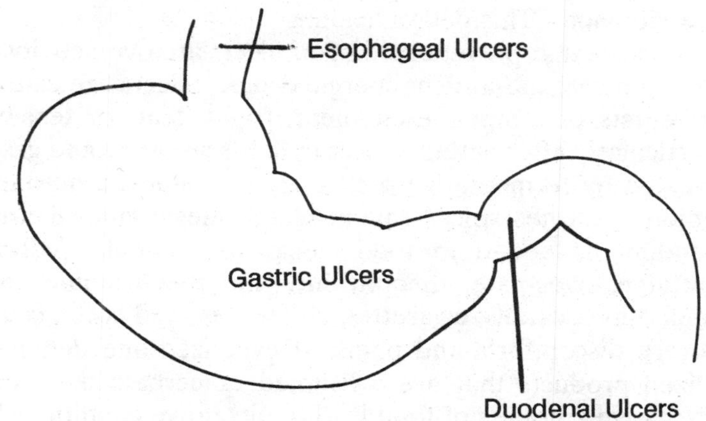

Figure 5. Illustration showing locations of peptic ulcers.

The word "peptic" refers to pepsin, a protein-digesting enzyme secreted by the lining wall of the stomach. Any ulcer occurring in the lower portion of the gullet (esophagus), the stomach, or the duodenum (a small portion of the small intestine connected to the exit of the stomach) is called a peptic ulcer.

The stomach and intestines are coated internally with a velvety type of very thin cellular lining called mucous membrane, which contains the secretory glands of the digestive juices. This membrane also absorbs food and protects the stomach muscle layers. The digestive juices in the lining would digest and erode the membrane itself were it not for the thick, firmly adherent layer of mucus that covers the internal walls of the stomach.

An ulcer is the erosion of the mucous membrane and is actually the result of the stomach's digesting its own tissue. Once started, the condition is aggravated, complicated, and sustained by the pepsin and hydrochloric acid secreted by the stomach. This delays healing.

Factors that prevent healing of ulcers are overactivity of the stomach and anticholinergic drugs. Ulcers are caused by bursts of temper, excitement, fright, fear, or tension, particularly after eating. Ulcer irritants are acids and gases created by fermentative processes, hot peppers, mustard, onions, radishes, spices, salt, ketchup, vinegar, and all other condiments added to food. Aspirin, alcohol, nicotine, caffeine, chocolate, theophylline, and theobromine contained in cocktails, cigarettes, coffee, tea, and cocoa cause severe discomforts and pains. Devitalized and demineralized products that are consumed exacerbate the ulcer. Excessive amounts of food lead to ulcerative conditions by causing an increase in the flow of digestive juices, which irritates the stomach lining.

Other foods involved in the causation of ulcers are flesh foods, which contain high quantities of nucleic and uric acids, and many other toxic substances. They produce high levels of toxicity in, and change the composition of, the blood. White sugar and white flour products and all drugs tremendously raise the level of poisons in the tissues and bloodstream, enabling erosion of tissues to occur more easily. Overeating of even the best foods may also produce ulcerative conditions. The effects of overeating, indigestion, flatulence, etc., always result in putrefaction of food, thus poisoning every cell in the body. Because they are irritants, iron supplements should be avoided if you have a gastric ulcer.

Dr. Gross states that the treatment for ulcers is to rest the digestive organs completely by fasting for seven to ten days. This will prevent the flow of the stomach acids and the aggravating peristaltic movements. (See natural hygienists under Resources.) A subsequent diet of delicate vegetables, fruits, and nuts, correctly combined, yields wonderful results. (Food must be chewed extremely well, at least 40 times each mouthful, because it is imperative that the food is well masticated and insalivated.) Gross has had several patients in various age groups recover completely from gastric and duodenal ulcers in every state of severity, using fasting and hygienic nutritional regimes. Given the chance, gastric and duodenal ulcers are the fastest-healing wounds in the body.

Dr. Gross concludes that the antacid powders and milk-cream advocated by physicians are abominations, for they cause further elaboration of acid gastric juice. They neutralize stomach acid at first but then backfire. Their calcium content promotes the secretion of gastrin, a hormone that triggers the release of more acid. Furthermore, the milk-cream causes clogging of the liver and gallbladder, preventing healing.

Vitamins A and C and zinc help heal ulcers. Foods with those nutrients are listed under Colitis.

It is a myth that ulcer patients should eat six times a day. In actuality, this is the worst thing for the stomach, because the stomach releases digestive acids whenever food enters it. Frequent feedings stimulate gastric acid secretion.

Stomach Ulcers

Duodenal ulcers and gastric ulcers have, basically, similar causative factors.

Both gastric and duodenal ulcers can be caused by, in addition to the usual nutritional or metabolic causes, severe nervous and mental stress. For any treatment to be successful, the psychological causes must be solved or removed.

In an acute case of active ulcers, whole grains, nuts, and whole-grain breads and cereals should be omitted from the diet, although cooked millet is beneficial. Sweet fruits can be eaten in moderation, and ripe bananas are well tolerated. All other fruits must be omitted for the first two weeks. Avocados are acceptable. All fried foods must be eliminated. Heated vegetable oils can be a contributing factor in developing ulcers. Also, soft drinks and sugar must be avoided. Do not eat or drink foods that are hot or cold; foods at room or body temperature are preferable.

For duodenal ulcers, take raw, freshly made cabbage juice, half a glass several times a day. For variety, mix 50-50 with carrot or celery juice. Raw potatoes are also recommended.

For stomach ulcers, take predominantly potato juice with a small amount of cabbage juice, half a glass several times a day on an empty stomach.

All juice must be freshly made and consumed *immediately* to get the full nutritive value from it.

MONOMEALS FOR EASY DIGESTION

Dr. Herbert M. Shelton stated that the eating of complex mixtures of foods is not seen in nature. Animals not only stay strictly with the foods to which they are constitutionally adapted, but they refrain from mixing these indiscriminately. The carnivore confines his meal to flesh; he never mixes his flesh with potatoes or fruit. The opossum, which eats flesh foods but is very fond of persimmons, does not mix these foods.

Man mixes his foods from all sources. He will combine in one meal the diet of the tiger (carnivore), that of the pig (omnivore), that of the sheep (herbivore), that of the bird (graminivore), and that of the primate (frugivore), and expect such a combination of foods to be as speedily and efficiently digested in his stomach as in the stomachs of the aforementioned animals.

The meals of man, until very recent times, have been very simple and have consisted of but two or three articles of food. With several notable exceptions, even the meals of the wealthy classes have been very simple when compared to the eating practices of today.

Shelton tells of Thomas J. Allen, M.D., early in this century, who gained a wide reputation as an advocate of the monomeal. He based his practice upon the discovery by Pavlov that each particular food requires for its digestion the secretion of a particular digestive fluid. He asserted that he had "demonstrated absolutely" that "cancer is due to a multiplex diet" and that the monodiet is the "physical factor in the cure."

Allen insisted that mixing foods different in character disorganizes digestion and nutrition. He did permit, though, a "rational combination" of "harmonious foods."

Shelton concludes that those who eat monomeals have much in their favor. The human digestive tract can make a far more complete and efficient adjustment of its secretions to the character of the food eaten if but one food is eaten at a time.

Remember that the more variety of foods at a meal, the more likely you are to overeat, as each food item stimulates the appetite with its own unique taste sensation. You may feel quite satisfied; yet, if another food is introduced, your appetite is once again aroused.

The monomeal is the most easily and efficiently digested meal you can eat. The only way you can get indigestion from a monomeal is to eat too much, to eat food contrary to your digestive capabilities, or to eat when stressed and fatigued. Of course, eating when not hungry is always a no-no!

The monomeal is recommended for breakfast because of the great ease with which a single food can be digested. Thus, the body's digestive system is not taxed, and its energy is not wasted on complicated digestive tasks. Also, the body receives the maximum nutrition from foods when they're eaten alone. It is the best guide we have that allows us to distinguish between the true demands of hunger and the misleading pull of appetite.

It really is doubtful that we need a wide variety of foods at any one meal in order to get all the talked-about essential nutrients. Many people do not realize that most fruits are a complete bill of fare and are replete with all the nutrients we need. Some tropical tribes practically subsist on monodiets of bananas, while others live almost exclusively on cassava. There are many fruits that are complete, well-rounded nutrient packages, notably grapes, bananas, figs, etc. Many of our simian cousins live on a quite restricted diet and still manage to grow, be strong and active, and live out their lives with minimal evidence of disease and aging.

Almost any food natural to the human palate is a complete food in itself, furnishing most, if not all, of our nutrient requirements. The body anticipates and prepares for future needs and emergencies, and if it does not get all that it requires in one meal, it will get it in the next meal or the one thereafter.

More likely our seeming need for wider variety merely reflects the general restlessness with which most of us are beset. As Herbert Shelton said, "Variety is the spice of gluttony."

However, natural hygienists do not advocate going on a monodiet for extended time periods, but simply want to demonstrate the point that the superior foods to which we are adapted provide a broader range of the nutrients we need than most of us realize.

The healthier you are, the easier it will be to control your thinking and recondition yourself to a sane way of living. The more physically healthy you become, the less effort it takes to control your emotions. The reverse is also true; the more control you have over your emotions, the more physically healthy you will become. It works both ways.

-- Dr. Vivian V. Vetrano, 1988

FIBER AND OUR DIET

T.C. Fry has observed that dietary fiber is being touted as a miracle substance that will prevent constipation, diabetes, bowel cancer, and many other disorders. More and more products on the market are boasting of their "high fiber content" by adding wheat bran and cellulose from wood pulp. And yet about 90% of our population still suffers from constipation. How can they be constipated, considering the increased amount of "high-fiber" packaged foods being consumed?

First of all, fiber does not help bowel movements; our peristaltic nerves and muscles are the prime movers of the bowels. If the intestinal tract is paralyzed or nonfunctional, no amount of fiber is going to induce it to work.

Fiber does tie up some toxic material in the intestinal tract so that the nerves and muscles are assaulted less by toxic alcohols, vinegars, and putrefactive by-products resulting from atrocious dietary practices. Otherwise, fiber is not necessary in the diet.

Fiber actually damages the alimentary canal. Bran is a food fragment; that is, it is only part of the whole wheat berry. It has many sharp edges that irritate and cut the delicate tissues within the gastrointestinal tract.

If we were to remove the natural fiber in fruits and vegetables by juicing and straining, bowel movements would continue, but not as copiously.

We need only observe and compare the bowel movements of a nursing infant, whose diet contains no fiber, to those of most adults who use fiber.

A healthy elimination pattern requires the bulk and fiber available only from a proper vegetarian diet. Vegetables, fruits, and whole grains, in contrast to meat, retain moisture and bind bulk for easy passage.

According to present research, natural fiber may be a significant deterrent to constipation, appendicitis, diverticulitis, cancer of the colon, heart disease, and obesity.

It is not the *presence of fiber* in a diet that is responsible for a scarcity of certain diseases, but the *lack of toxic substances* in the diet. For example, toxic materials such as refined flours, refined sugars, preservatives, condiments, etc., are abundant in the diet of Americans.

BUT WHERE DO I GET MY PROTEIN?

Protein is the most complex of all food elements, and its assimilation and utilization are the most complicated.

Protein is not any more or less important than any of the other constituents of food. They all play a crucial role in making a food a food and are used together synergistically.

Americans are under the delusion that they get their proteins from meat, eggs, and milk products. But the truth is that Americans get little if any of their amino acids from these sources even though they eat abundantly of these "food" categories. When meat is cooked, the protein of the meat coagulates, and much of it deaminates. Thus, it becomes relatively void of usable nutrients. But even if meat is eaten raw, humans have insufficient hydrochloric acid to digest it properly.

Proteins are in every cell of every living substance. Every *natural* food contains proteins, which, by digestive processes, are reduced to amino acids. The word "natural" means food *natural* to the human physiological disposition and foods in their raw state. It is important to note that the body absorbs and uses *only* amino acids, not proteins. The usable amino acid content found in plant life is far in excess of that to be found in flesh foods.

Human amino acid requirements are very low, perhaps only 10 to 25 grams per day. But the average American eats 105 grams a day, most of it cooked and unusable. Consuming more than the body requires places a heavy burden on the system as it tries to rid itself of this excess. The excess protein not only robs you of your energy but is bacterially converted to toxic materials such as ammonia, hydrogen sulfide, mercaptans, skatols, putrescine, and indoles.

If you are eating protein for the purpose of gaining strength, you are defeating the purpose. The strongest animals in the world do not eat animal flesh for strength; elephants, oxen, horses, and gorillas eat leafy matter, grass, and fruit.

Where does the average person get usable amino acids? From fruits and vegetables. In fruits, people get all their nutrients in fairly "predigested" form. Fruit "proteins" come to us as readily absorbable amino acids.

Some examples of protein content in fruits and vegetables are the banana and the pear, which each provide 1 gram; a stalk of broccoli, 6 grams; an avocado, 4 grams; a carrot, 1 gram; a half cup of almonds, 13 grams.

Proteins are in every living food. You can't find a single living food that doesn't have protein. Our illnesses are caused not by lack of protein *but by too much protein*. Proteins in excess of bodily needs putrefy, especially when proteins are cooked, deranging them beyond usability.

The only ways to become deficient in protein are either to starve or to eat foods that contain no protein (sugar and oil). If a person eats enough food to maintain near normal weight, and if a variety of whole foods is eaten, a protein deficiency is impossible.

There are a total of 23 amino acids that the body utilizes. There are *eight amino acids* that the body must appropriate from outside sources. The body can make the fifteen others from the eight if necessary. There are many fruits and vegetables that contain all eight of the amino acids not produced by the body: carrots, bananas, Brussels sprouts, cabbage, cauliflower, corn, cucumbers, eggplant, kale, okra, peas, potatoes, summer squash, sweet potatoes, and tomatoes. Also, all nuts and sunflower and sesame seeds contain all eight.

It is not necessary to combine lower-quality proteins together at each meal so that one protein makes up for the deficiencies in the other protein, because the body maintains a large pool of the subunits of protein, the amino acids. If a protein is eaten that is too low in certain amino acids, the body can supplement the need from its reservoir of amino acids and make this protein relatively complete and usable.

LACK OF VITAMIN B-12 AND STOMACH DISORDERS

Some people believe vegetarians are deficient in B_{12} as a result of eating fruits and vegetables exclusively, but almost no natural food has vitamin B_{12} in it. There is no vitamin B_{12} in grass either, yet cattle have plenty of vitamin B_{12}. We humans get our vitamin B_{12} the same way other animals do: from by-products of bacterial activity in our intestinal tract. Also, certain other B-complex vitamins are created in and absorbed from the intestinal tract.

Major factors in B_{12} deficiency are stomach diseases that interfere with production of the essential bacterial activity and intestinal disease that interferes with normal absorption of B_{12}. The use of alcohol, tobacco, and drugs such as neomycin and oral contraceptives may increase loss of B_{12} from the body.

HELP FOR OVEREATING

We must eat to live, not live to eat.

-- Fielding

Victoria BidWell, the author of *The Health Seekers' Yearbook*, offers the following suggestions.*

Overeating is a symptom of compulsive behavior, and it is antithetical to calm awareness, both emotionally and physiologically. The overeater can practice behavior modifications to increase his awareness of his eating habits.

Two conditions are important prior to using the behaviors. *First, eat at designated eating areas only*. When people use every room in the house and at work for eating, each room unconsciously becomes a stimulus to eat.

Secondly, *eat as a separate activity*. People eat more food than they normally would when they distract themselves with other activity. Such examples are watching TV, reading, driving, telephoning, writing letters, etc. With the exception of pleasant conversation, no extraneous activity should distract the diner from every bite he takes. The heightened awareness is what breaks the addiction.

BidWell suggests nine simple behavior modifiers to slow down the eating process and increase awareness. Psychologists say it takes 21 days to break a long-term

---

*This material is compliments of Victoria BidWell and GetWell * StayWell, America! See Recommended Reading for details to receive GetWell's **free**, 150-page catalog.

compulsive habit. The best time to start is TODAY! Mark your calendar, and just do it one day at a time.

1. Rest in a quiet room ten minutes before eating. Eating at a high level of anxiety induces uncontrollable eating.
2. Take at least 20 minutes to eat. Avoid snacks and plan three meals a day. Place a timer before you and pace yourself. It takes about 20 minutes for the physiology to signal the hypothalamus that enough food has been consumed.
3. Put utensil (or food, if no utensil) down between bites. This action is the best, if you use no other. **LET GO OF THE FORK!** Take time to chew and swallow. (I might add that the best part about eating is the taste and the pleasing aromas.) Relax, take a deep breath.
4. Take smaller bites. This mechanical behavior slows down eating.
5. Use a napkin between bites as another short circuit to prevent the reflex action of the loaded fork going to your mouth.
6. Stop for three minutes during the meal. Doing so will give you a feeling of control over the attraction between you and your food. The harder taking three minutes is for you, the higher your state of anxiety, the more you need the time to gain control of your eating.
7. Leave a small amount of food on the plate. This is a difficult exercise for many people, since most of us have been raised to "eat everything on your plate." More harm will come from overeating than from throwing away food. To leave a little food is to show yourself that you are in control.
8. Leave the table when finished. The table is a designated eating area. You have to leave the table eventually -- let it be NOW!
9. If possible, rest after each meal. Even sitting or lying down for five minutes aids digestion. And doing so

continues the composure gained during the meal. Take a few minutes, also, to congratulate yourself on having eaten yet another meal with controlled awareness.

Victoria BidWell says that compulsiveness and composure are opposite emotional events, with opposite physiological parameters. They cannot be experienced simultaneously. If the food addict nurtures composure, the diner need not eat compulsively ever again.

EXERCISE TO ELIMINATE STRESS

Mike Benton, director of the American College of Health Science, offers a stress-management program of exercise, diet, and relaxation.

1. Exercise is your best friend in combating stress because exercise channels the excess energy created by stress into a natural and positive outlet.
2. By following a natural hygiene regimen of fresh fruits, vegetables, nuts, seeds, and sprouts you will have a superabundance of all needed nutrients, including B vitamins as well as important minerals and trace elements that build strong bones.

On the other hand, junk foods, refined sugars and starches, processed foods, non-foods like alcohol and coffee, and many of the other substandard foods eaten deplete the body of B vitamins, which are the very nutrients your body needs to withstand stress.

The stress-junk-food cycle starts with eating a sugary, comforting food, such as pastry or candy. After the food is eaten, additional B vitamins and other nutrients are depleted. The nutrient loss predisposes the nervous system to more stress attacks, and more junk food is eaten.

Food, or digestion, is also used to deaden the feelings of stress. When the body is loaded down with a mass of food to digest, the mind becomes cloudy, dull, and desensitized. The food is used as a drug to obliterate feelings of tension, depression, despondency, or stress.

3. The opposite of stress is relaxation. Learn to alternate periods of stress with periods of relaxation.

HOW TO BREAK A BAD HABIT

Who is strong? He that can conquer bad habits!

-- Ben Franklin, 1770

Habit is habit and not to be flung out the window by anyone . . . but coaxed down the stairs, one step at a time.

-- Mark Twain, 1870

Dr. Ralph Cinque, in an article for *Healthful Living* (January 1987, p. 14), suggested ways to overcome bad habits such as smoking cigarettes, drinking coffee, or eating junk food. It is a step-by-step plan that does not depend upon total abstinence, does not cost any money, and does not require outside help.

Habits are acquired patterns of behavior. We are born into this world without any habits at all. All habits are acquired, cultivated. This is equally true both of good habits and bad habits.

Choose what is best; habit will soon render it agreeable and easy.

-- Pythagoras

One approach to unlearning destructive behaviors is the same as to learn a constructive one -- systematically. Use a mechanized plan, executed one step at a time.

The first step to breaking a bad habit is to acknowledge your desire to quit and to cultivate an attitude of avoidance. For instance, instead of saying to yourself, "I can never eat ice cream again," you should say, "From now on, I will avoid eating ice cream." Avoidance may be a more reasonable and worthwhile goal than strict abstinence because it is more attainable. The first principle for behavior modification should be: *Don't set yourself up for failure*.

The second step is to rid your home of the harmful foods. This step is crucial because home is where most of our habits are built and maintained.

Cinque concludes: aim as high as you can, but don't punish yourself if you fall short of it. Never stop trying; every day you have a new opportunity to take charge of your life.

Dr. William Esser says that the best way to break wrong eating habits is first to wipe the slate clean. This is done by fasting, which is remarkable for dislodging deeply ingrained habits. The sense of taste, which has been dulled by long use of hot and cold foods, by highly seasoned foods, and by the paralyzing alcohol, coffee, tea, etc., needs rest and regeneration, which the fast provides. A supervised fast will be carefully broken and foods gradually introduced in proper amounts and combinations. A full appreciation for the fine flavors in well-grown natural foods is readily developed under these conditions, and natural foods will normally appeal far more than poor-quality, deficient conventional foods.

T.C. Fry further suggests a fast of 3 to 7 days. Then break the fast on freshly squeezed juices the next day. Thereafter, partake of mostly raw fruits with some vegetables. Nuts and seeds must be slowly incorporated into the diet after a week. The fast and correct diet will help you free yourself of the body pollution that weighs you down and saps your willpower.

The secret to getting rid of old, destructive habits lies in loving and respecting yourself so much that you do not succumb to the addictive stimulation that is so powerfully projected to make us puppets on the strings of Madison Avenue manipulators.

-- Jo Willard, 1982

HOW TO GO ON A WEEKEND FAST

I humbled my soul with fasting.

-- Psalm 69:10

Scientists who have studied fasting have found that a forty year old man can be fasted for 3 weeks and be restored to the physiological level of a 17 year old! Now that is remarkable! Where else can you find anything which will restore youthfulness? There is nothing else in all the realm of nature that can accomplish this as can fasting.

-- Dr. David J. Scott, 1980

If the medical professionals courageously popularized the fast among their patients, there would be infinitely less suffering than there is now. That many would be saved who now die through the drug and feeding treatment is a certainty.

-- Gandhi, 1945

Because of the many time pressures most of us are under, fasting is becoming a luxury. But if we don't voluntarily take the time out to regain our health, we will be forced to lie in bed when the condition becomes acute.

Mike Benton, the director of the American College of Health Science, has suggested a program for a weekend fast in an article written in *Healthful Living* (April 1982, p. 34).

Benton suggests starting a fast on Friday afternoon and continuing until late Monday. Of course, even better is a three-day holiday weekend. Fasts that are 72 hours in length are remarkably effective in rejuvenating the body and may be safely undertaken without supervision (provided you are not taking large doses of medicine).

A weekend fast may be safely done in the home, where you will be free from mental stress and social demands. Let your friends and family know that you will be unavailable for the weekend. Use a sunny room for your retreat. Remove the phone and television from the room. Have a pitcher of distilled water handy, since this is all you will be drinking.

If the home is not conducive to a fast, you might consider going to a motel or on a camping trip.

It is not necessary to take an enema or purgative before or during the fast. You can give your fast a head start by eliminating sugar, alcohol, processed foods, meat, coffee, and dairy foods from your diet as soon as you possibly can. On Thursday, eat only raw fruits and vegetables. Do not use oil or vinegar in your salads.

On Friday morning, start the day with freshly made juice or a few pieces of fruit. Eat a raw vegetable salad for lunch. (See lunch ideas under Brown Bagging It, in the Recipes section.) Have your last meal about 3 p.m. You'll know your body is detoxifying when your tongue becomes white-coated and your breath is very foul.

On Saturday, sip some distilled water through the day to avoid dehydration, but only when you are truly thirsty. Drink room-temperature water, but if you prefer to drink it body temperature, it's acceptable to do so.

If you have enough energy, take a short walk. If the weather allows, sit in the sunshine and fresh air as much as possible.

You might experience a headache or nausea late in the day. This is a positive sign that your body is detoxifying.

By Sunday, you will have a sour taste in your mouth, and your urine may be very dark with a strong odor. If you don't have a bowel movement while fasting, don't worry about it; it will come after you break the fast. Don't enervate the body with enemas, and most definitely do not take any laxatives. (That in effect will end the fast along with detoxification. Ed.)

Don't be alarmed if you feel weaker or worse today than you did Saturday. By now your body will be pouring old toxins out for elimination, and these poisons may occasion temporary discomfort and distress. Take a warm bath in the evening and relax.

By Monday, you probably will not feel the pangs of hunger on arising. If you feel very hungry by lunchtime, then it's time to break the fast. When you break the fast, follow this procedure:

For your first meal, eat one to three pieces of fresh, juicy fruits such as oranges, apples, grapes, or melon slices. Eat only one type and a small quantity. Chew very, very slowly and thoroughly.

Wait two or three hours for your next meal and follow the same procedure. Continue this through the day.

On Tuesday, you can eat fresh fruits and raw salads. Wait until Wednesday before introducing other foods besides raw fruits and vegetables into the diet.

After the fast, your body may react uncomfortably to substandard or "junk" foods. Listen to your body and stay away from these "foods."

A weekend fast can be successfully undertaken once a month to allow for gradual detoxification. If you eat a high-quality diet between times, each fast will become more effective than the last.

T.C. Fry's book *Fasting: Fastest Way to Vibrant Health* is available on Order Form #2. Paul C. Bragg's book *The Miracle of Fasting* can be found in health-food stores.

The one sure road to better nutrition and better health is first to fast. Let your body do its professional and expert job of nourishing you during the fast, and then, with your taste buds cleansed of the false craving for junk, you will readily embrace the fresh fruits, vegetables, nuts and seeds and you can finally break away from the junk.

-- Seneca, 62 A.D.

WHAT TO EXPECT WHEN YOU IMPROVE YOUR DIET

Remarkable things begin to happen to the body and mind when you improve your diet. The amazing intelligence present in every cell of the body is heightened. The rule may be stated thus: when the food coming into the body is of higher quality than the elements present in body tissues, the body begins to discard the lower-grade materials to make room for the superior materials, which it uses to make new and healthier tissue.

Furthermore, live-food eaters have more energy, need less sleep but have more energy, are more alert, and think more clearly. Live food eaters are less subject to stresses and nervous tensions than conventional eaters.

Overweight people who undertake the eating of live foods, especially in conjunction with an exercise regimen, experience a drastic weight reduction.

Best of all, live food eaters become virtually sickness-free!

"Withdrawal" Symptoms Follow Use of Improved Diet

What are the symptoms or signs which become evident when we first begin to omit the lower-grade foods and introduce superior foods? Example: when the use of a toxic stimulant such as coffee, tea, chocolate, or cocoa is stopped, headaches are common, and a letdown occurs. This is due to the discarding by the body of the toxins caffeine and theobromine, which are removed from the tissues and transported through the bloodstream to the eliminating organs. When the blood circulates through the brain during its many bodily rounds before the noxious agents reach their final destination for elimination, these irritants register in our consciousness as pain. Other signs of body detoxification are discomfort along the spine due to its concentration of nerve cells.

The most frequent symptom is bloating of the system. The cleansing ability of fruits and leafy vegetables will stir up accumulated toxic waste, creating gas and bloat. Usually, this bloating passes within 48 hours. On rare occasions, it may last 72 hours. Don't be alarmed if the bloating causes you to add two or three pounds during the first few days. The body is simply adjusting itself for the task ahead.

You may feel exhausted or anxious. You may experience diarrhea-like symptoms, but do not be alarmed. This is a positive effect. The cleansing aspect of fruit and leafy vegetables washes impacted fecal matter from the intestinal walls and flushes it out of the system in this manner. Soon you'll feel light and renewed. It is imperative that you do not use a product like Kaopectate to stop this detoxification process. To stop the elimination would retain the waste in your system. Loose stools rarely last more than two days. Rest and allow the body to do the work it was designed for. As the toxins in your system are stirred up, you will experience some nausea.

It is likely that you would have a discharge of mucus from your nasal passages. This is not a head cold. Again, your body is spewing out the excess toxins that have been built up and stored in the mucous membrane.

To avoid uncomfortable symptoms, introduce raw foods into the diet slowly. Start by replacing one of your normal meals each day with a raw one. Drinking fresh-squeezed orange juice in the morning will give you a natural mental high lasting several hours. Gradually eliminate meat and processed foods from your diet until you reach a balance of about 75% raw and 25% cooked. At this point, you will discover the benefits of raw food.

Some programs that should be employed when your body is going through detoxification symptoms are the use of massages, exercising, jogging, walking, sun baths, skin brushing, therapeutic baths,* and jumping on a rebounder (trampoline).

But once we become aware of the impact of our food choices, we can never really forget. For the earth itself will remind us, as will our children and the animals and the forests and the sky and the rivers -- that we

---

*Instructions on skin brushing and therapeutic baths are at the end of this section.

are part of this earth, and it is part of us. All things are deeply connected, and so the choices we make in our daily lives have enormous influence, not only on our own health and vitality -- but also on the lives of other beings, and indeed on the destiny of life on earth.

-- John Robbins, 1988

FOODS TO ELIMINATE COMPLETELY FROM YOUR DIET

Salt, **sugar** (it weakens the immune system), **pepper**, **spicy seasonings**, **candy**, **chocolate**, **syrup**, **MSG**, **garlic**, **condiments**, **commercial dips**.

Vinegar and all products using vinegar, such as **pickles** and **pigs' feet**.

Alcohol, **cocoa**, **coffee**, **tea** (some herb teas are acceptable), **carbonated beverages**, **canned and pasteurized juices**, **artificial fruit juices**.

Pasteurized milk and all products made from it, **ice cream**, **whipped toppings**, **nondairy coffee creamer**.

Lobster, **clams**, **oysters**, **shrimp** (the sea scavengers, which feed upon the wastes of other fish); **all fish**.

White flour products, **hulless grains**, **pasta**, **crackers**, **snack foods**, **white rice**, **cold cereals**, **pizza**.

All red meat, **hot dogs**, **bologna**, **bacon**, **sausage**, **liver**, **luncheon meats**.

All roasted and/or salted seeds and nuts; **peanuts**.

All lard and shortening and margarines made with **hydrogenated oils.**

All canned and creamed soups; anything canned.

All fried foods, potato chips, snacks, popcorn,* pretzels.

Curry dishes, Szechuan cooking, enchiladas.

BUT I STILL HAVE INDIGESTION!

On occasion, when you begin to eat fruit, and even if you are following all the instructions in the book, you may still experience flatulence. The main reason this happens is that there is an accumulation of food debris and body wastes that have built up over the years and encrusted the lining of the stomach and intestines. Fruit has a tendency to loosen these impacted wastes. Then they are ejected from the intestines. In the process of loosening this matter, gases develop in the intestinal tract. Most people don't experience this situation, but some who are particularly toxic will experience it for two to three weeks. Overall, even though it's an annoying problem, it's positive evidence that the cause of the problem is being eliminated.

You may also experience an initial bloating of the system. Usually this bloating passes in 48 hours, but it can last as long as 72. Do not be alarmed if you add a few pounds during the first few days. It is simply the body adjusting to physical changes. You might experience symptoms similar to diarrhea, but this is only the body ridding itself of toxic waste, and no attempt should be made to stop this process. Other symptoms of detoxification are

---

*An outright carcinogen due to the high heat required to pop it.

body aches, headaches, exhaustion, anxiety, insomnia, and nausea. That is why it is best to start this program over a long weekend holiday.

Even on a transitional diet -- part raw, part old diet -- you may experience these symptoms for weeks or months, simply indicating that the body is going through a cleansing process. Every individual is different. For instance, people who have taken drugs (prescription or not) on a regular basis are more apt to experience some temporary discomfort than are non-drug users.

DRY BRUSH MASSAGE INSTRUCTIONS

Dry brushing of your skin will revitalize and increase the eliminative capacity of your skin and help throw toxins out of the system. Skin brushing also stimulates and increases blood circulation in all underlying organs and tissues.

Normally, when not overloaded with toxins, the body has the ability to cleanse itself through a large group of specially designed organs, glands, and transportation systems: alimentary canal, kidneys, liver, lungs, skin, lymphatic system, mucous membranes of various cavities, etc. But the largest eliminative organ is the skin.

Uric acid, the main metabolic waste product and a normal component of urine, is found in perspiration. If skin pores become clogged with dead cells, uric acid and other impurities will put a strain on the other eliminative organs, mainly the liver and kidneys, by increasing their detoxification load. This causes overworked organs, which will eventually weaken and become diseased.

The best brush for a skin massage is a natural-bristle brush with a long handle so you can reach all parts of your body. They are sold in health food/supply stores. Buy a brush that is soft if you have delicate skin. My skin is very sensitive, so I use a soft-bristle garment brush. If you do

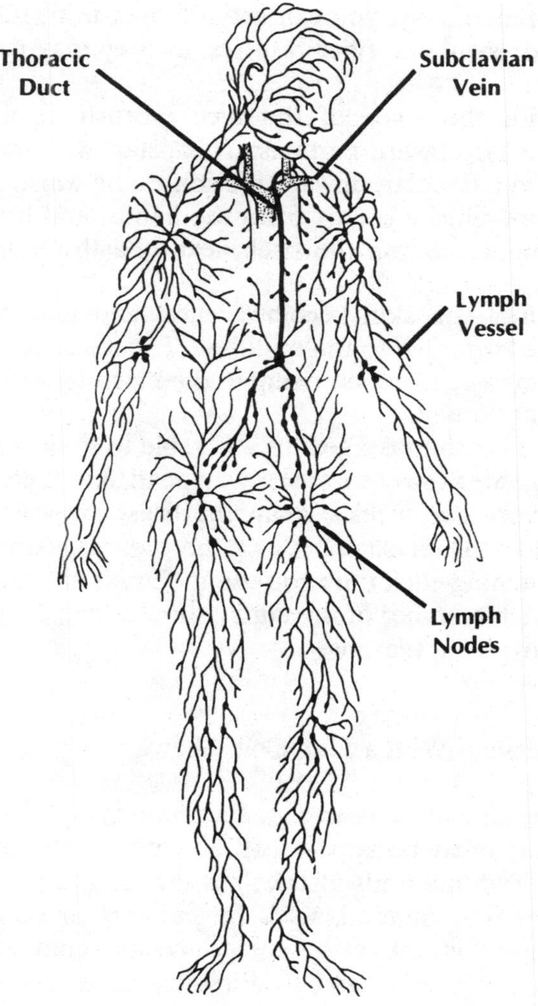

The Lymphatic System

not have a brush and wish to start your dry brush massage program immediately, you can use a loofah mitt. Do not use nylon or synthetic fiber brushes, as they may damage the skin.

Start with the soles of the feet. Brush vigorously, making circular upward motions. Next, start with the feet, and brush in a circular, upward motion to the waist. After both feet are finished, start from the hands, and brush to the breastbone. Brush the back next. Lastly, brush the neck.

Brush until the skin becomes warm and glowing. It should take from five to ten minutes. The ideal time for a dry brush massage is upon rising in the morning and again before going to bed.

After the brush massage, it is advisable to shower or rub down with a wet towel to wash away dead skin flakes.

Once every two weeks, clean the brush by washing it with a mild soap or shampoo, or the old, dry skin flakes will cause itching each time you use it. Dry it in the sun on its side. Each member of the family should have a separate brush for hygienic reasons.

Follow Massage With a Hot/Cold Shower

Skin brushing loosens up copious amounts of dead layers of skin that must be washed off for the brushing to be effective. Two methods of taking a shower are presented here. The first method, used by patients in European health clinics, is the alternating hot and cold shower, followed by dry brush massage. First, take a hot shower for three minutes, or until you feel warmed up; then take a cold shower for about ten to twenty seconds. Repeat this three times, ending with cold water. After the shower, rub yourself dry with a coarse towel and then give yourself a brush massage until you are thoroughly warmed up.

The second method, which is suitable for relatively healthy people, is to take the dry brush massage first and finish with alternating hot and cold showers, then drying and warming up with a coarse towel.

The alternating hot-and-cold shower has a beneficial and stimulating effect on all the vital functions of the body, especially on the glandular activity.

THE BIOMECHANICS OF SQUATTING

This chapter was contributed *by Dr. William F. Welles, a chiropractor who practices applied kinesiology and nutrition. (See Resources for more information.)*

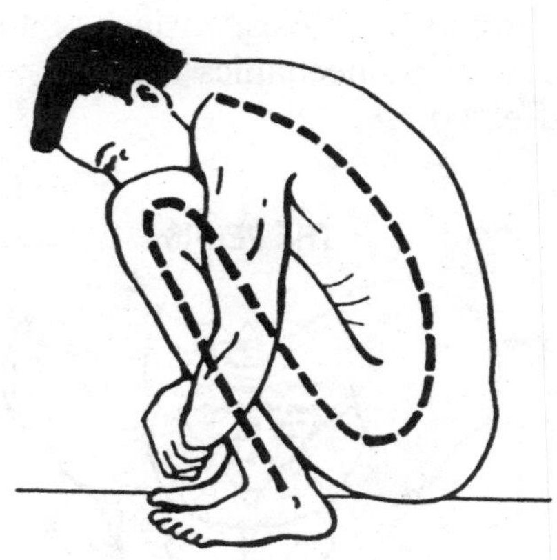

Squatting is the most central posture known to humanity. Throughout history people have always squatted. It is the most common posture used by "uncivilized cultures" in sitting, and is our only option as a posture of elimination in natural surroundings. In the squatting posture, muscles are magnificently stretched, structural balance is maintained, and our energy and bowel circuits are activated. Western civilization's adoption of the sitting posture, especially during elimination, has robbed its citizens of structural balance and energy flow. In China, if individuals cannot squat flat-footed on the ground, they are considered sick. If this standard is correct, the majority of adult people in Western society are ill. Suffice to say, the use of the modern-day toilet is the beginning of disease. When people use the toilet, they suffer from incomplete elimination.

When an individual cannot squat, it is because the muscles of the lower extremity and pelvis have become foreshortened and imbalanced. The muscle groups most foreshortened from lack of squatting are the erector spinae, adductor, hamstring, calf, and the external rotators of the pelvis. This foreshortening leaves an individual with a condition known as "abunosis," or lack of a rear end. More importantly, the biomechanics of the whole body are negatively affected.

THE PELVIS

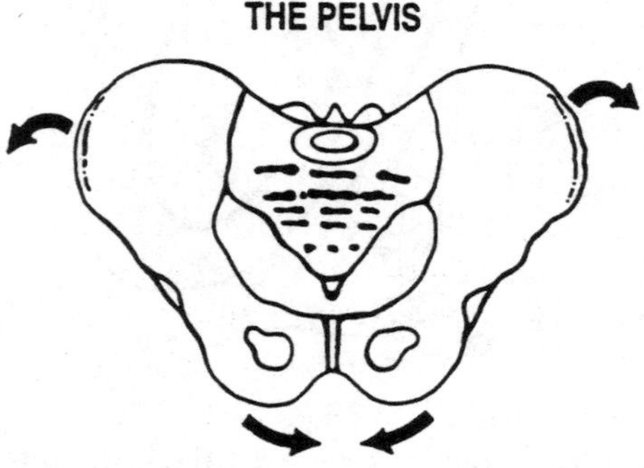

Tight calves cause the muscles that support the arch to turn off, and a pronated foot results. The dysfunctional foot then causes knee and low back instability. Tight adductor, hamstring, and external rotators in the pelvis, such as the piriformis, cause the buttocks to be sucked under. When this happens, the ilia flare outward and the ischiums come toward the midline (see diagram above). The phenomenon can be confirmed by palpating for tension in the piriformis muscles and feeling for spasms in the sacroiliac ligaments. Such flaring out of the ilia and shifting of the ischiums dramatically compromises the structural balance of an individual and predisposes him or her toward low back and sacroiliac problems.

As though this were not enough, when we make use of the modern toilet, further structural imbalances occur according to the following scenario. When be bear down without the support that is normally afforded by the thighs while squatting, we make demands on the ileocecal valve beyond its capacity. The valve therefore becomes dysfunctional, allowing fecal contents to travel backwards into the small intestine; when that happens, those digestive contents infect other organs with fecal bacteria. Oftentimes the first organ to go is the liver, as I have talked about in my book, *The Shocking Truth About Cholesterol*. The liver is our oil filter. It is an in-line oil filter between the gut and all the rest of the organs and the bloodstream. When we have a backup of our plumbing, the liver is the first organ to get infected and the pancreas is next in line. These organs are infected directly from the gut via ducts or pathways from the organ entering into the intestinal tract.

Because bearing down without support is so stressful to the system, the abdominal and psoas muscles in the lower right quadrant weaken. I see this muscle imbalance pattern in approximately 80% of my new patients on a postural analyzer. The pattern is evidenced by the right buttock rotating toward the posterior and the torso shifting off the center line to the left.

Structurally, the right ilium then lacks support and flares more outward. This is evident when the right buttock is palpated for tenderness, especially at the crest of the ilium.

That the sacroiliac joint is distressed is also evident by the tenderness of its ligaments.

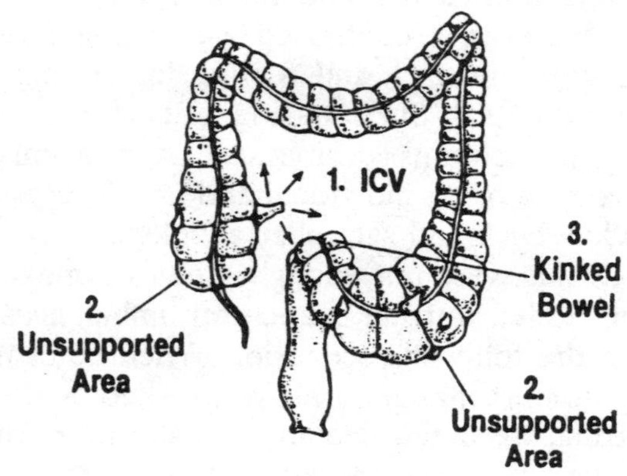

When the right psoas weakens, the lumbar spine twists, negatively impacting the lumbar discs. There is no more important muscle to balance in the case of disc problems than the psoas. Furthermore, when there is a weakness in any given part of the body, reactive tightening always occurs elsewhere. In this case, when the right psoas is weak, the left psoas usually tightens, as does the lower bowel on the left. This produces a stricture in the bowel and backs up plumbing like a clogged drain.

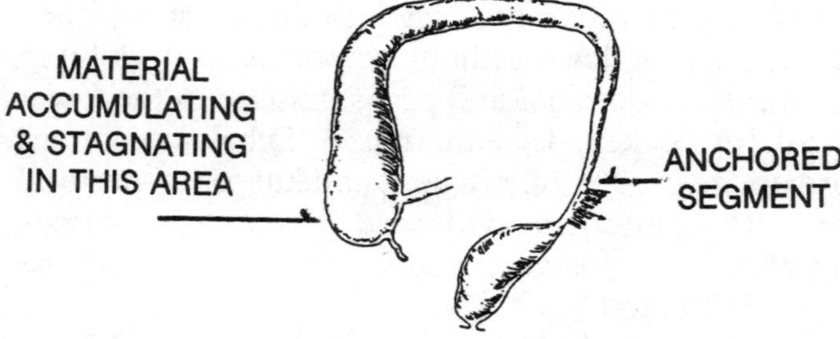

Above is a picture from a book called *The Prevention of Diseases Peculiar to Civilization*. Sir Arbuthnot Lane, a structure-oriented surgeon, operated on thousands of bowels, and found a strictured area in the lower left quadrant in virtually all of them. He stated that this blockage, which I see as reactive tightening secondary to a dysfunctional ileocecal valve, robs us of our health. He went on to say that cancer results from autointoxication secondary to this dysfunctional bowel. He urges us to return to the standard of a bowel movement after every meal established by Hippocrates 2400 years ago. This standard is supported by the relatively recent physiological discovery of the gastrocolic and duodenocolic reflexes.

Many great chiropractors such as Dr. Cox and Dr. Goodheart have pointed out the strong correlation between bowel problems and low back pain. It is interesting to note that the associated point for the bowel is located at L5, the most involved lumbar vertebra. The majority of cases of low back pain that I treat respond very favorably when chiropractic and bowel reflex therapy are used together. I have all my clients squat, but stress it more when they have low back pain.

When the pelvis's balance has been warped by foreshortened and weakened muscles secondary to lack of squatting and use of the toilet, its function is very much compromised. Normal craniosacral respiratory motion is grossly inhibited. The benefit of normalizing craniosacral motion on such individuals is at best transitory.

When an individual adopts the squatting posture in elimination, the ileocecal valve normalizes, and elimination improves. In this way, the right psoas and lower abdominal wall are strengthened. This then allows the bowel to function better, thus improving the state of the lower lumbars.

When the same individual also squats as an exercise, *dramatic* benefits are achieved. Squatting gradually normalizes pelvic geometry so that spinal energy is increased. Adjusting a pelvis like this back into position is not plausible; however, chiropractic adjustments greatly facilitate this wonderful change.

When the pelvis is balanced, cerebrospinal fluid flows once again as normal craniosacral movement is reinitiated. The cerebrospinal fluid is the lifeblood of the nervous system. When it is flowing well, spinal adjustments carry far greater impact. All organs of the body profit from renewed life currents.

The squatting posture also stimulates the tibialis anterior, which affects stomach 36 and 37. Stomach 36 is the major energizer of all the meridians in the body, filling them with increased life force. Stomach 37 is the major bowel point, and dramatically improves bowel function.

The benefits of squatting are so great that the late Dr. Randolph Stone likened his three squatting postures to an acre of diamonds in everyone's back yard. He stated that squatting "is literally riding the River of Life's energy waves and tuning into them!"

While it is necessary to squat in the act of elimination, this is not enough to regain normal elimination and good health. We need to assume the squatting posture and stretch the calves and hamstrings *daily* to lengthen muscles that involve the function of the bowels.

Using the Welles Wedges to Squat

If squatting causes strain to the muscles, the Welles Wedges (on Catalog Sheet #1) will comfortably help you stretch your muscles. The test for determining whether you need a wedge under your feet for squatting exercises is as follows:

1. Use a carpeted area with no obstructions for six feet.
2. While bare-footed, try to accomplish the squatting postures shown on the next page.
3. While squatting, rock forward and back one inch.
4. If you can't accomplish these postures without the feeling of falling backward, then you need the Welles Wedges.

These are very powerful exercises, and you are asking the body to make profound changes to muscles in a state of imbalance for years. To realize the maximum benefit, start doing these postures one at a time and for a short duration. The higher up on the wedge you need to put your heels, the more foreshortened your muscles are, and the more conservative you should be. These exercises produce the most dramatic health benefits imaginable, by opening up the pelvis. Follow the directions to the letter so as not to injure yourself and rob yourself of the rewards of squatting.

Note: for further stretching of the calf and hamstring muscles, turn the Welles Wedges with the narrowest side under your heel.

Schedule

Do leg warm-up exercises before you practice squatting exercises.

Day 8 (after one week of calf and hamstring stretching): Do Exercise #1, the General Squat, for 20 seconds.

Day 9: Add Exercise #2, the Abductor Squat, for 20 seconds.

Day 10: Add Exercise #3, the Adductor Squat, for 20 seconds.

Day 11: Add on 10 seconds to each exercise, up to one minute each (approximately Day 16).

CAUTION: Individuals with a history of low back, hip, or knee pain should consult with their health care practitioner before starting these exercises. If you experience any knee or other joint problems, stop the exercises for a couple of days and consult your physician.

Exercise #1: General Squat

1. Position the blocks approximately 9 inches apart in front and 6 inches apart in the back.

2. Squat on the blocks with the heels just high enough to rock forward and back 2 inches freely.

3. With armpits over knees, rock forward and back gently for 60 seconds.

4. Then move side to side and rotate, each for 20 seconds.

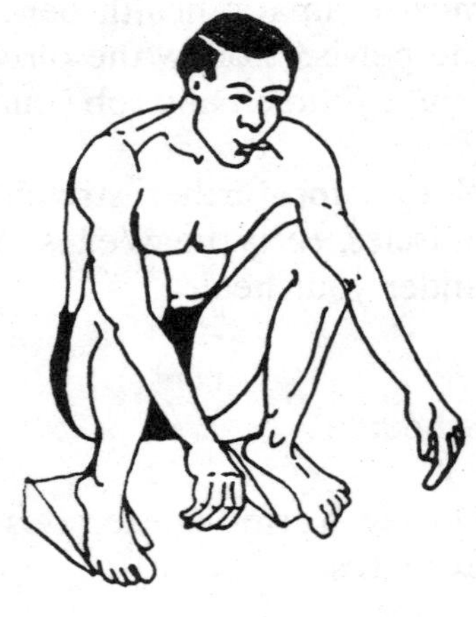

General Squat

Exercise #2: Abductor Squat

1. Feet in the same position, move arms outside knees, interlacing your hand around opposite wrist (heels may need to be higher).

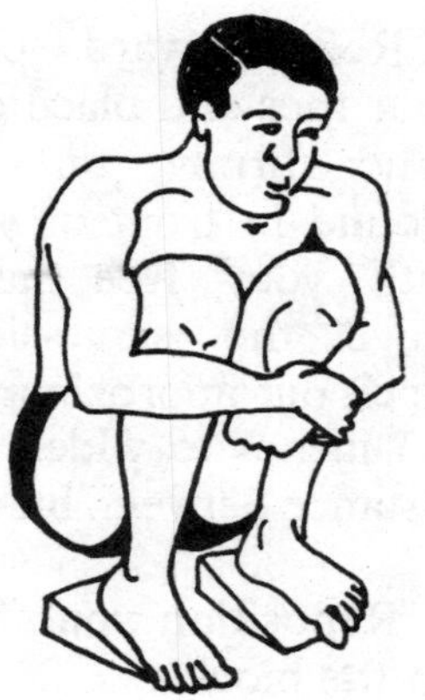

Abductor Squat

2. Gently pull your legs together approximately one inch; don't overstrain.

3. Rock forward and back as before for one minute.

4. Then move side to side and rotate, each for 20 seconds.

5. When moving from side to side, you can rotate your abdomen within your thighs. This movement has the most powerful positive effect on the male and female sexual organs. Prostate and premature ejaculation problems in males, and PMS and other sexual dysfunctions in females, can improve dramatically!

Exercise #3: Adductor Squat

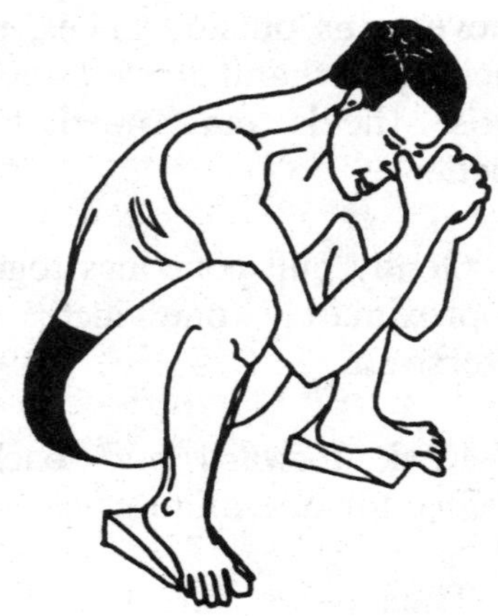

Adductor Squat

1. Roll forward onto your toes and place one hand firmly on the ground in front of you; with your free hand, move the same-sided block out approximately 2-3 inches to widen the distance between blocks.

2. Reposition your foot on the block.

3. Bring your arms inside your knees and bend your elbows; with one hand inside the other, place thumbs on juncture between nose and eyebrows; treat tender points found here with light pressure.

4. Gently stretch your thighs outward one inch and rock forward and back for one minute.

5. Then move side to side and rotate, each for 15 seconds.

Note: when getting up from these positions, roll forward onto your hands and knees and then stand up slowly.

The Benefits of a Slant Board

It's a scientific fact: your entire existence on this planet is dominated by the Law of Gravity. This universal force, whether you acknowledge it or not, is constantly pulling your body out of shape. Reclining your body with your feet above your heart and your heart below your head naturally reverses the pull of gravity on your face, neck, back, organs, and legs.

Examples of the many consequences of not living compatibly with gravity and Newtonian Law are found everywhere. Gravity's ceaseless drag on the body contributes to sagging abdomens, prolapsed organs, varicose veins, leg ulcers, mental fatigue, drooping shoulders, sagging buttocks, reduced height, bulged-out midsections, and deep facial wrinkles.

In addition, if you sit and stand all day, then sleep with your head propped on a pillow all night, gravity decreases the flow of blood to your head. Poor circulation to your brain, scalp, complexion, gums, eyes, and ears usually adversely affects their functioning.

Because we spend our working hours standing or sitting upright, gravity is constantly pulling downward on our muscles, blood, organs, and other parts of our bodies. That's why people's feet ache and become swollen. Their back muscles tense, and they become tired and irritable.

With a little effort, you can do something to reduce the effects of the earth's mighty magnet. You can make gravity your friend and use its strength and pull for a reverse uplifting effect.

You can reverse all of the aforementioned conditions with a slant board. When you come home from work, lie on it for 15 minutes, with your feet elevated. This takes the strain off your muscles and your heart and gets things back into position where they belong. You'll find it very relaxing and probably the most pleasant 15 minutes of your day.

The slant board is especially beneficial because it helps replace the internal organs that have become lowered or displaced. In many persons, the internal organs are pushed from their normal position by part of the large intestine that is often filled with accumulated wastes. The slant board exercises will improve digestion, help establish normal regularity, and help restore the organs to their proper position, particularly the prolapsed organs.

The daily use of a slant board increases the flow of blood into the head and brain area. The importance of getting blood into all the extremities cannot be emphasized too much. The brain is the center of our living; all movements emanate from the brain first, and if the brain is blood-starved, we naturally have slow reactions in other parts of the body.

Experts have compared slant board benefits to improvements gained from the yoga head and shoulder-stand. The positions reverse gravity's pull and stimulate all body processes. Digestion is improved; constipation and varicose veins are relieved; the nervous system is toned; the aging process is slowed, the brain stimulated, the facial tissues and cells rejuvenated.

In addition to all the physical benefits the slant board brings, it also relieves mental anxiety and induces peaceful relaxation.

You can easily make a slant board with plywood, hinges, foam, vinyl covering, 14" legs, and a leather strap. The strap is for holding your feet down when you do pull-ups. If you are a small person, you can use an ironing board covered with a blanket. You can also raise the foot of the bed (for all-night sleeping) with 6", 8", or 10" blocks of wood. Perhaps you can start with the shorter height and slowly increase to the higher height, giving your body time to acclimate to the change.

If you wish to invest in a regular slant board, one is available from Dr. Welles. His book, *A New Slant on How to Flatten Your Abdomen*, is included. Victoria BidWell also offers a slant board. The boards can be ordered on Catalog Sheet #1 at the end of this book.

REFLEXOLOGY

From a neighbor who is a reflexologist, I learned first hand how helpful the method can be when suffering from the discomforts of indigestion. An excruciating stomach pain that I had all morning was gone after only a half hour of massaging certain parts of my feet.

Reflexology is a form of therapeutic foot massage which facilitates healing by improving circulation and nerve function.

The feet are a perfect microcosm of the body. All the nerves at the soles of the feet are connected to all the organs in the body. When pressure is applied to certain points on the feet, electrochemical nerve impulses are activated, forming a "message" to a specific organ.

Reflexology is considered to be a holistic healing technique which aims to treat the individual as a whole in order to induce a state of balance and harmony in body, mind, and spirit. The reflexologist doesn't cure -- only the body has the capacity to cure. What reflexology does is work with the subtle energy flows that revitalize the body so that its own natural healing ability can initiate healing.*

---

*See books under Recommended Reading, and Reflexologists under Resources.

To Calm an Upset Stomach

The stomach reflexes are located in the soft area just in front of the thumb, a little below the web. Massage this area with the thumb of the opposite hand, using a press and pull motion, until the discomfort is gone.

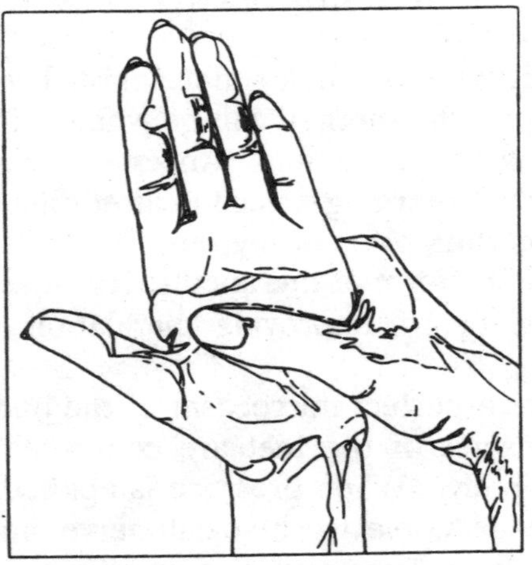

Figure 6. Stomach reflex point.

HOT WATER BOTTLE

When experiencing an upset stomach, a very soothing and helpful treatment is a hot water bottle. Don't use boiling water -- just hot water. Leave the bottle on as long as you like.

A super king size hot water bottle can be ordered on Catalog Sheet #3 at the end of the book.

AN APPEAL

The best service a book can render you is, to impart truth, but to make you think it out for yourself.

-- Elbert Hubbard

All of the diseases mentioned in this book, which are common in industrialized countries, are virtually unknown in developing countries. But when these countries adopt the diet and lifestyle of Western civilization, they develop the same diseases.

Apparently you have are concerned about your eating habits, or you would not be reading this book. Interestingly, all condiments, pickles, hot peppers, etc., because of their overpowering toxicity, would instinctively be rejected by a baby. But little by little we have developed a taste for these items. Now that you have seen the harm they are doing to you, you should make a drastic change in your dietary habits. Give up harsh condiments, and be assured that, although you may not enjoy your food at first, nature will soon slough off the jaded taste buds and restore your normal sensitivity. You will once again appreciate the delicious flavors with which nature has imbued her foods.

Don't expect the result of a lifetime of harmful eating habits to turn around overnight. Depending on the degree of damage your wrong eating habits have caused, it may take several years for your health to return fully.

Once you have read this book, you no longer have the defense similar to that which cancerous smokers use -- "We weren't told how dangerous smoking was." Herbert M. Shelton said, **"You had these perversions because of ignorance and conditioning, but now you know that every transgression you commit upon your body exacts its toll such that you suffer to some measure, whether you're aware of it or not. Your body does not always make you**

consciously aware of the problems your bad habits impose upon it. When your eating habits develop into irreversible diseases, you'll have only yourself to blame."

Life is full of trade-offs. We can either make the commitment to eat properly or have the medical industry take charge of our lives. The latter means having our bodies drugged, being cut open to have our vital organs removed, or enduring the devastating effects of radiation.

You are herewith presented with an opportunity to enhance your life greatly. Do you have the fortitude and resolve to carry out its mandate?

Ancient wisdom tells us that when the student is ready, the teacher appears. The lessons we need come to us when we're ready to learn them. Often, they come through other people. The teachers in our lives don't usually instruct us directly, with lectures or coaching. Instead, we learn from our relationships or experiences. Sometimes a teacher appears when we least expect it. We may be worrying about a problem, and suddenly find a book containing exactly the information we need. We may feel we are all alone in the world, and suddenly meet someone who seems to understand us completely.

Our readiness is an important factor in our learning process. Being ready means being open and continuing to take one step at a time, one day at a time.

-- Author Unknown

Part III
Recipes

INTRODUCTION TO RECIPES

The menus presented in this book contain only two compromises: the use of a tiny amount of *real butter* (raw, if you can get it), and the minimum amount of virgin olive oil to make sauces. There are no "meat substitutes" in these recipes. If eating meat is immoral (and unhealthy), so is the lust for eating it.

One of the most important parts of any diet is the salad. A large salad of uncooked vegetables should be taken with each protein and each starch meal. Leafy green vegetables are the cleansers of the digestive system. They have bulk, an abundance of nutrients and minerals, and chlorophyll (nature's healer). Obviously, I am not referring to the typical salads such as egg salad, potato salad, shrimp salad, and the like, served in restaurants or delicatessens. Their dressings and/or vinegar cause digestive problems. My salad dressings are made from fresh vegetables.

You'll recall that digestive leukocytosis develops when cooked food is eaten, but this does not happen if raw food is eaten before or with a cooked meal. That is why, in all of my Transition Recipes, I have always included raw vegetables with the dish.

There are no so-called desserts in the recipes. Besides always being wrong combinations with all the other foods in the meal, they contribute to overeating, thus undermine health. If you must have fruits, skip everything else. Fruits are all-dessert meals.

A short fast is helpful before starting a raw vegetarian diet or to start new, improved eating habits like eliminating dairy products. During a fast, the entire eating pattern is broken, acclimatizing the body to change.

You can expect some difficulty in making the transition from highly seasoned foods to simple foods, but you will experience immediate rewards with higher energy levels, a cleaner digestive system, increased mental clarity, and sweeter body scent. You'll also find that you can solve life's many problems with greater facility, and you will not find many incidents as stressful.

Don't make your change in diet a source of anxiety for yourself or those around you, especially at mealtime. Your meals should be an enjoyable experience. A serene atmosphere, both outside yourself and within, is of primary importance for good digestion.

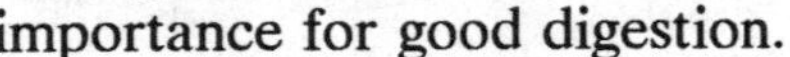

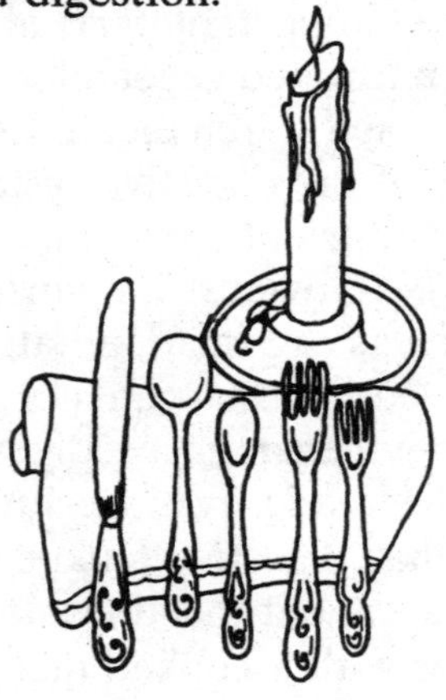

Make dining a gracious event; put out your finest china, colorful placemats, a flower arrangement, with soft music in the background. Try to present a treat instead of a treatment to minimize the change of food habits.

Discuss the day's problems calmly when you come home from work or an hour after dinner, but never at the dinner table. Instruct the children that squabbling at the dinner table will not be tolerated. Any negativity at the dinner table is harmful to *everyone* dining.

If eliminating harmful foods from your diet seems like a Herculean task, I suggest that you eliminate the worst items first. For the first week, commit yourself to do this for one week. Then take it one day at a time. By the end of the week, your body will accustom itself to the improvement. Then follow the same commitment for each of the next four weeks. Eliminate these items the first week (of course, any item you can, as long as you make any attempt to do so):

Vinegar and all products containing it
Red meat
White refined flour

The second week, eliminate these items:

Seasonings
Milk and milk products
Sugar

The third week, eliminate these items:

Alcohol
Coffee
Tea
Soda pop

By the fourth week, you will no longer have a craving for these health-destroying foods, because the live food gives your body all the required nutrients it needs to function physically and mentally. Enjoy your transition from conventional food faddism to a back-to-nature diet.

Initially, you may think it takes more time to prepare raw foods than to cook conventional meals. But once you get the knack of it, it takes the same amount of time. The real time is saved in cleaning the utensils. Actually, more time is gained because you will have more mental and physical energy. Less time is wasted in recuperating from harmful eating practices.

Specifics About Food Combining

Nuts and Seeds

Concentrated foods such as nuts and seeds should be eaten with or as part of a vegetable salad. The water content of the salad vegetables offsets the lack of water in nuts and seeds.

Nuts and seeds are protein-fat foods. Fats are slow to digest, and their presence with protein makes nuts particularly slow-digesting. Delayed digestion encourages fermentation and putrefaction. This results in the formation of gas and toxic materials that give rise to the many discomforts of indigestion.

After eating nuts, three hours should elapse before eating fruit.

Fruit

Fruit is the only food that requires no digestion in the stomach. It contains its own digestive enzymes and, when ripe, is virtually predigested. Any delay in the movement of sugars from the mouth into the intestines results in their fermenting. The by-products of fermentation are toxic and disease-producing. This is why fruit should *never* be eaten with or immediately following any other food. It is essential that you eat fruit on an empty stomach.

Fruit contains all of the necessary nutrients required by your body sustaining life. That includes glucose from carbohydrates for energy, as well as vitamins, minerals, fatty acids, and amino acids for building protein.

Only fresh fruit should be eaten. There is no benefit in eating fruit that has been processed or altered in any way by heat. The body can utilize fruit only in its natural state. Cooking destroys its nutrients.

Fruit should never be eaten with proteins because fruit acids inhibit the secretion of hydrochloric acid and thus interfere with protein digestion. Do not combine fruit with any vegetable except lettuce and celery. It is best not to combine fruits with vegetables (especially cooked vegetables), proteins, or starches, because if such a combination of foods is eaten, the digestion of the fruit will be delayed and subject to fermentation.

Bananas, if not properly ripened, may present a sugar/starch combination that may not properly digest.

Dried Fruits

Dried sweet fruits should be used sparingly. Use but one kind at a meal, in small amounts. They should be combined only with sweet fruit and/or with lettuce and/or celery.

Citrus Fruits

Citrus fruits are best eaten at monomeals or at bimeals of oranges with grapefruits, pineapple, strawberries, etc. They should never be combined with starches such as breads, pastas, grains, potatoes, carrots, beets, squash, peanuts, etc. Nor should they be combined with proteins, except with nuts or seeds.

Melons

Melons comprise an additional class of fruit, as they decompose even faster than other fruits. They are more than 90% liquid and leave the stomach quickly. If melons are eaten with other foods, even fruits, they will ferment in the stomach. Regarding melons: eat them alone or leave them alone.

Tomatoes

Tomatoes should not be combined with starchy vegetables or proteins except nuts, seeds, and avocados. They do not combine well with starches because the enzyme ptyalin is needed in the digestive juices for breaking down the starch, and the acid in the tomato destroys ptyalin.

Lettuce and Celery

Fruits, except melons, may be combined with either lettuce or celery. These vegetables are neutral in digestive chemistry, and they enhance digestion of the fruits, especially the concentrated, sweet varieties. Lettuce is an extremely nutritious vegetable. Because lettuce is high in water content, it is an excellent combination with more concentrated foods of lower water content such as pecans, sunflower seeds, walnuts, sesame seeds, filberts, and pignolias (pine nuts).

Sprouts with Fruits

All fruits go well with sprouts since the starch in the seeds has largely been converted to the simple sugars that are also found in fruits. Protein in sprouts has been converted to amino acids, and as such is predigested.

Sweet Potatoes

Sweet potatoes are another typical sugar/starch combination that may end in gassy episodes for some people.

Legumes

All legumes should be soaked at least three hours or overnight to activate the enzymes in them; otherwise, they are indigestible.

Important Information About Foods

Butter Versus Margarine

During World War II, butter was not available, so a synthetic substitute, margarine, was created to take its place. Margarine is made by turning "pure liquid polyunsaturated oil" into a solid bar of grease. The liquid is turned solid by hydrogenation: hydrogen gas is bubbled through the oil until it solidifies.

Margarine is touted as having less fat, being lower in calories, and providing some protection against heart disease. The truth is that butter and margarine have the *same* number of calories and contain the same amount of fat, but margarine *will contribute* to the very problems commercials imply it will prevent, particularly heart disease!

I have used butter in some of my recipes, but I have put restrictions of only one pat per person per meal.

Oil

Natural hygienists advocate avoiding all fats except those that occur naturally in seeds, nuts, and avocados. Natural oil in the diet is an essential nutrient. Heat-pressed oils are rancid, and the chemical substances produced irritate the delicate linings of the stomach and intestines. Prolonged use of rancid oils has a carcinogenic effect on the human body. Also, rancid oils destroy vitamins E, F (essential fatty acids), A, and carotene that may be present in the body when the oil is consumed.

You may think that cold-pressed oils are acceptable, but the so-called cold pressing of oils is a misnomer, as it is simply a description of the process of extracting oil under low heat. Either a hydraulic press or an expeller (screw-type press) is used to extract oil. Heat during processing can reach between 130° and 150° F.

The only oil I recommend using is double virgin olive oil. It is the first oil to come out of the rollers in the processing of olives. Use only the smallest amount necessary.

Eating Desserts

Desserts such as cakes, pies, puddings, ice cream, and stewed fruits, eaten at the end of the meal, combine poorly with vegetable or protein meals and cause indigestion. Eaten on top of meals, they lie heavily in the stomach, requiring no digestion there, and ferment. Bacteria turn them into alcohols, vinegars, and acetic acids. Also, chances are that the eater has already eaten to capacity, making it unnecessary to consume more food. Desserts serve no useful purpose and are not advisable. Regarding desserts: DESERT THE DESSERTS!

Instructions for Recipes

How to Soak Garbanzo Beans (Also Known as Chick Peas)

Place dry garbanzo beans in a wide-mouth jar or covered casserole dish. Use a proportion of one part beans to three parts water. Always use distilled water. Put in refrigerator and shake the jar occasionally. The beans will triple in size. Shaking prevents the beans from pressing against each other when they swell, making it difficult to get them out of the jar. Rinse and change the water after the first day. Soak them for two days.

How to Steam Vegetables

For those uninitiated to the eating of raw foods, I have provided some recipes in which the main ingredient is steamed but accompanied by raw food. As your body and attitude become acclimated to this change, you will notice that the vegetables taste overcooked, and each time you steam them, you will be inclined to lessen the cooking time.

Place a cup to a cup and a quarter (depending on the size of the pot) of water in a pot. The water should be below the level of the steamer to prevent the loss of nutrients. Bring to a boil. Place vegetables in the steamer, cover the pot and lower heat to keep the water *simmering*. The temperature of the water and steam stays the same

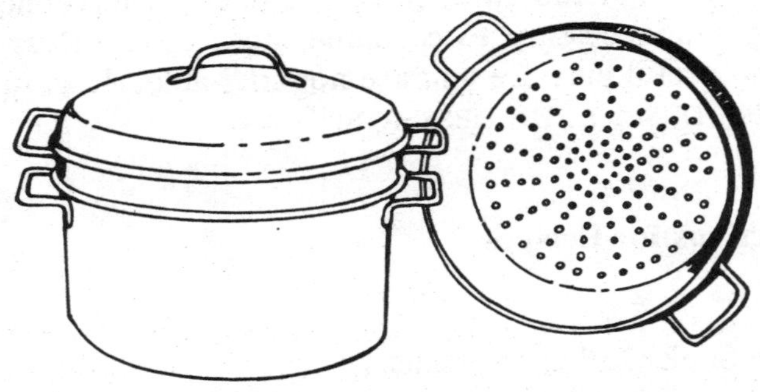

regardless of how rapidly the water boils! The color that you see in the water and the odor you smell when food is being cooked evidence a loss of vitamins and minerals and the destruction of enzymes. At 120° F, the enzymes (which are valuable amino acids) are destroyed.

Steaming time varies with the age of the vegetable. Week-old cauliflower and broccoli take less time to steam than when they are fresh.

How to Clean Vegetables

Wash fruits and vegetables thoroughly before you eat them. I use a product from Amway called LOC. Put one teaspoonful per gallon of water in a basin or sink. There are other commercial fruit and vegetable cleaners on the market. Wash fruits and vegetables with a vegetable brush when applicable. Don't leave fruit in water; wash it quickly, or rotting will occur. Don't wash peaches until you're ready to use them, or they will rot. The same advice applies to asparagus and Brussels sprouts. Use a spray bottle of LOC for this purpose. Never soak vegetables for more than a few minutes. Rinse thoroughly and dry with a dish towel.

When storing tomatoes, use a cloth napkin to prevent them from touching. They will rot where they touch. Wrap cucumbers, zucchini, spinach, and lettuce in cloth napkins or dish towels; they will stay fresh longer.

How to Kernel Corn

Place a large bowl in the sink. Move a corn kerneler in a twisting motion over the corn cob while squeezing the kerneler tightly. When you have gone halfway down, switch hand positions and continue to the end. Go firmly and slowly toward the end, keeping the corn facing the bowl because the kerneler will "snap" when it reaches the end, causing the corn to scatter. Tap the kerneler clean over the bowl. Using a paring knife in a firm downward motion, scrape the "cream" off the cob into the bowl.

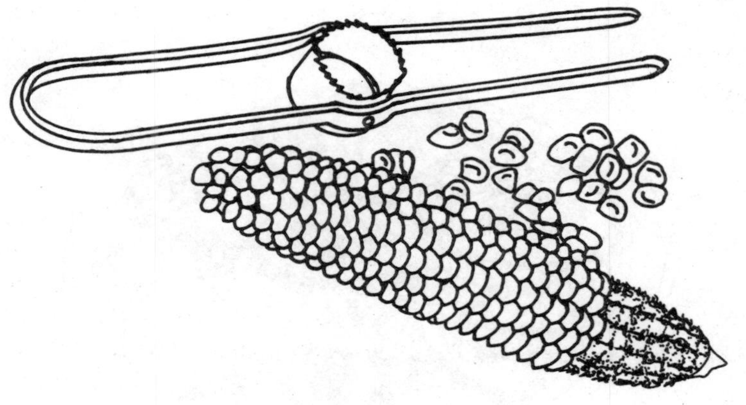

Raw Food and Saving on Utility Bills

The average family in America can save from $10 to $12 per month on utility bills by switching to a raw food diet. Imagine the reduction of fossil fuel used nationally if this were done!

The cooking of meat and the use of oils in frying create an estimated 200 pounds of airborne grease per household that is released in the home every year. In fact, airborne grease is more carcinogenic than cigarette smoke! Some grease may go out the stove exhaust flue, but much is left to coat the walls, cupboards, drapes, floors, windows, window fans, screens, furniture, hair, skin, and nasal passages. Compounding this problem is the use of polluting chemicals to remove the grease periodically.

The time saved by not doing the extra cleaning of these items can be better used for productive purposes.

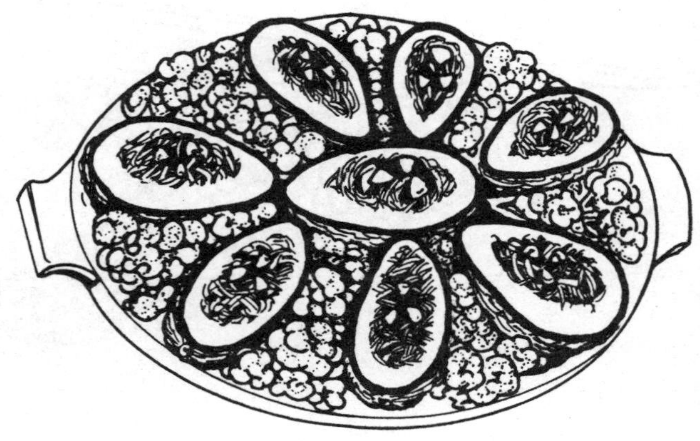

Kitchen Utensils You Will Need

Electric food processor or grater

Manual food grater/slicer

Electric food blender

Electric nut chopper/grinder

Hand-held slicer

Assortment of carbon steel knives

Oriental vegetable cleaver/chopper

Chopping board

Corn kerneler

Potato peeler

Julienne cutter (also known as a potato chipper)

Assortment of salad bowls

Measuring cups

Steamer

Digital timer

About Aluminum Cookware

Copper and aluminum cookware should not be used if the cooking surface itself is made from either of these metals. Acid foods cooked in aluminum interact with the metal to form aluminum salts, which are toxic. A letter to the *New England Journal of Medicine* points out the connection between aluminum and brain disorders such as dementia, Alzheimer's disease, behavior abnormalities, poor memory, and impaired visual-motor coordination. *One British study shows that aluminum cookware may cause indigestion, heartburn, flatulence, constipation, and headaches.* Pots and pans with nonstick finishes such as Teflon or Silverstone scratch easily and can contaminate food with bits of plastic while cooking is taking place.

Liquid Soy Products

I recommend using Bragg's Liquid Aminos because that particular soy product is not fermented. Also, I find all liquid soy products too salty-tasting. At first I diluted 1 cup of liquid soy with ¼ cup of distilled water. After a while, it was still too salty-tasting. I now dilute it half and half.

CONTENTS TO RECIPES

BROWN BAGGING IT

Almost one-third of all meals are eaten at workplaces or in restaurants. It would be detrimental to continue your harmful eating practices when at work. I have made up several menus that you can take to lunch. The first group is for unrefrigerated items. The second group must be taken in a cooler.

The ambience in restaurants is rarely pleasant. Diners are talking, dishes are clanking, cash registers are ringing. Peace and quiet would be beneficial to you physically and mentally at lunchtime. If you brought your own lunch, you could eat at a local park, outside on the green lawn, or even in your car if nothing else is available, so as to break the constant pressures of interacting with people all day.

You will actually get physical and mental energy from fresh fruits at break times throughout the day. Coffee may pick you up temporarily, but it causes mental retrogression after an hour or so. Fruit will give you a natural mental lift. Take no more than three kinds of fresh fruit in the same group or only one kind of dried fruit. Dried figs and dates should not be eaten at the same meal.

Keep a knife, fork, spoon, potato peeler, paper napkins, paper or plastic dishes, cloth napkins, toothpicks, and moist towelettes at work so that you won't have to be concerned about including them every time you pack your lunch.

Don't peel or slice anything until you are ready to eat. The food will lose some of its nutrients, and the open surfaces will begin to oxidize.

Brown Bag Lunches

Avocado, handful of well-scrubbed **Jerusalem artichokes**, several **plum tomatoes**, the tender parts of **celery**.

Avocado, several well-scrubbed **carrots**, fresh **string beans**.

Bananas, persimmon or **papaya, dates.**

Apples, kiwi, grapes, sprouts.

Cantaloupe, celery.

Cooler Lunches

Avocado, jicama, carrots. Cut, but don't peel, desired amount of jicama at home. Seal tightly with plastic wrap. When ready to eat, insert knife under edge on top and strip off. Cut into slices.

Almond butter, tender **celery stalks, broccoli florets.**

Almond butter, red bell pepper, jicama, sunflower sprouts.

Almond butter, **Chinese peas**, well-scrubbed **carrots.**

Spinach, **cauliflower florets**, **red** or **yellow bell pepper**, small jar of **Bragg's Liquid Aminos**. Tear spinach into bite-sized pieces. Chop pepper. Put all in dish and sprinkle with aminos.

Corn on the cob (remove husk at home), **string beans, carrots, dip.**
(Dip: prepare at home half of an unpeeled **zucchini**, 1 tablespoon **Bragg's Liquid Aminos**, 1 tablespoon **virgin olive oil**. Swirl in a nut chopper or blender.)

Baked potato (well scrubbed, baked the night before and refrigerated). **Red bell pepper**, **spinach**, **Bragg's Liquid Aminos**. When ready to eat, slice potato. Cut pepper in half and slice. Put on bed of spinach. Sprinkle with aminos.

Baked yam (well scrubbed, baked the night before and refrigerated), **spinach**, **corn on the cob**.

One-half head of **lettuce**, **carrots**, **Chinese peas** or **string beans**, small jar of **Bragg's Liquid Aminos**.

If you can find **yeast-free pita bread**, or any whole-grain/yeast-free bread, it would be acceptable. You can make **avocado**, **lettuce**, and **tomato** sandwiches. **Unsalted whole-grain crackers** could be used in place of the bread.

Lettuce, **almond butter**, **red** or **yellow bell pepper** (cut into strips), **sunflower sprouts**. Spread almond butter on lettuce. Put pepper and sprouts on top. Roll up and hold in place with toothpick.

Boston lettuce, **apples**, **grapes**, **raisins**, **sprouts**, **celery**.

Bananas, **blueberries**, **mango**. Prepare mango at home. Seal tightly with plastic wrap.

Plain **granola**, **celery**, **cucumber**, **string beans**, **lettuce**.

HORS D'OEUVRES

(always check your particular condition to see if you can have all of the ingredients)

Fruit Kebabs

CITRUS KEBAB

Chunks of **pineapple, orange** slices, **blackberries**, with slices of center section of **celery** or any part of **fennel** in between each fruit. Smash some of the blackberries and pour over top.

TART TREAT KEBAB

Chunks of **pineapple**, **kiwi**, and **strawberry**, with **blackberries** between each fruit. Liquefy plums or grapes and pour over top.

SUBACID FRUIT KEBAB

Apricot chunks, **mango** chunks, **cherries**. Puree some of the cherries in nut chopper or blender and pour over top.

SWEET FRUIT KEBAB

Sliced **banana, dates, persimmon**. Puree ½ cup pre-soaked **raisins** in nut chopper. Pour over top.

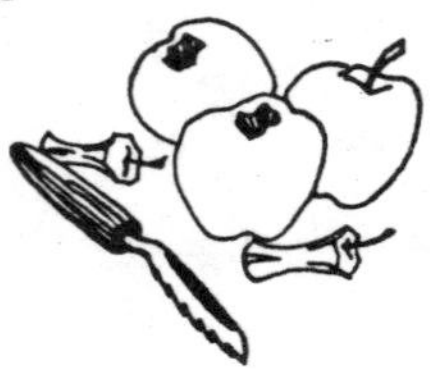

Apple Twist Kebab

Pour 2 cups of **organic apple juice** into a small bowl. Put all fruit into bowl as you cut it. Peel a **red apple** in one continuous peel. Cut apple, **pear**, and **plum** into chunks. Push only one end of apple peel on skewer (skin side first). Let hang. Slide fruit chunks on skewer. Twist apple peel around chunks of fruit and push end into skewer. Pour apple juice over top.

Salad Kebabs

Combine any of the following group on a skewer. Spoon any of the **dips** (listed in the next section) over the top.

Cauliflower florets, **cherry tomatoes**, folded **spinach** leaves.

Broccoli, **mushrooms**, **zucchini** slices, **red bell pepper**.

Zucchini slices, **snow peas** cut in 1" lengths, **red** and **yellow bell peppers**.

Green Crepes

Use soft lettuce leaves like Boston lettuce or red-leaf lettuce to roll up any of the combinations below:

Soften **avocado** with 2 tablespoons **pink grapefruit juice** and add fresh **corn**, grated **carrots**, and **sunflower sprouts**.

Grated **carrots**, chopped fresh **parsley**, **sunflower seeds**, finely chopped **celery**.

Diced **cucumber**, young **peas**, finely diced **tomatoes**.

Bean sprouts, raw **pepitas** (chopped), diced **cucumber**, fresh **parsley** (chopped).

One **zucchini** and **carrot**, finely shredded; **peas**.

Coarsely grated **jicama**, fresh **corn**, chopped **parsley** or **watercress**.

STUFFED FENNEL

Remove outer stems from **fennel**. Put 2 heaping tablespoons **almond butter** in nut chopper; add enough distilled water to soften. Remove from chopper and add diced **cucumber** and grated **carrot**. Sprinkle with chopped **alfalfa sprouts**.

STUFFED PEPPER STRIPS

Cut into quarters 1 **red** and 1 **yellow bell pepper**. Remove seeds. Put 1 cup sprouted **sunflower seeds** in nut chopper and chop slightly. In a separate bowl put ½ cup finely grated **carrots**; 1 small **avocado**, diced; ½ cup chopped **alfalfa sprouts**; and ½ cup finely diced **cucumber**. Mix well. Spoon onto peppers. Alternate the colors when placing on serving dish.

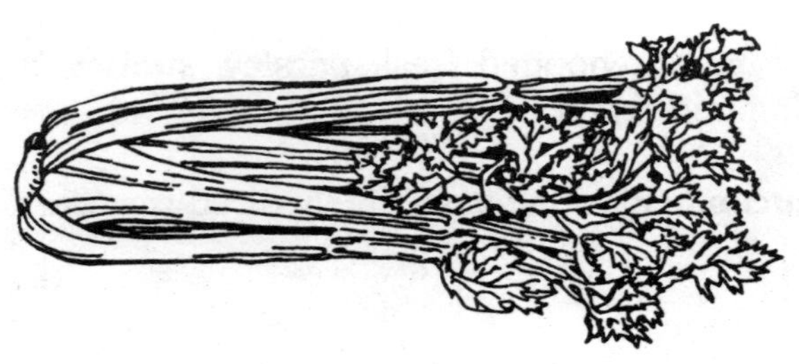

Stuffed Pepper with Jicama

2 large **yellow bell peppers**
1 cup grated **jicama**
1 ear **corn**, kerneled
2 **plum tomatoes**, diced
2 **plum tomatoes**, chopped, pureed
Bed of **greens**

Cut peppers in half from bottom to top. Leave stems on. Remove seeds.

Combine jicama, corn, and diced tomatoes. Put peppers on bed of lettuce or sprouts. Spoon mixture into peppers. Pour pureed tomatoes over top.

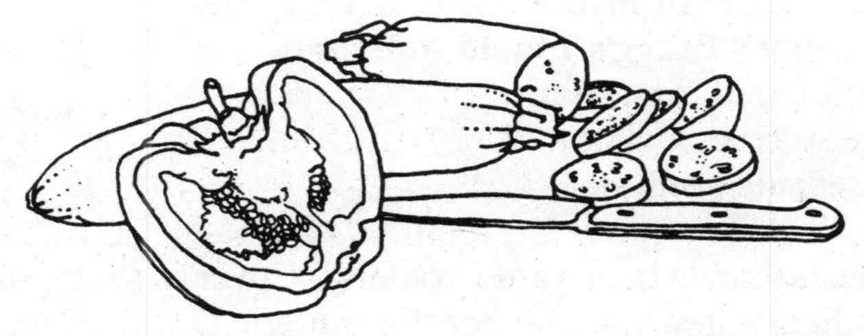

DIPS

CARROT & JICAMA DIP

½ medium **cucumber**, peeled and chopped
2 tablespoons **pink grapefruit juice**
1 cup finely shredded **carrot**
¼ cup coarsely ground **sunflower seeds**

Liquefy cucumber and grapefruit juice in an electric blender or a nut chopper. Put all ingredients in a small bowl and blend.

GARBANZO DIP*

¾ cup dry **garbanzo beans**, soaked (see "How to Soak Garbanzos" in Instructions for Recipes)
2 tablespoons **Bragg's Liquid Aminos**
¼ cup chopped **tomatillo**
⅛ cup **watercress**, chopped
¼ cup **sesame seed meal**

Rinse garbanzo beans after soaking. Cover in saucepan with distilled water and simmer 5 minutes. Drain. Grate in food processor. Put remaining ingredients in blender in order given. Grind until chunky.

*This dish requires soaking of garbanzo beans two days in advance.

GUACAMOLE

2 ripe **Haas avocados**
2 tablespoons **pink grapefruit juice**
1 medium-small **tomatillo**, finely diced
3-4 **plum tomatoes**, finely diced
¼ cup chopped **parsley** or **watercress**

Cut avocados in half lengthwise. Remove seeds and cut thin slices in both directions while still in skin. Scoop out pulp. Sprinkle with grapefruit juice and smash with a fork in a small bowl. Add tomatillo, tomatoes, and parsley. Mix. Serve with vegetable dippers.

KOHLRABI ITALIENNE

6-8 **kohlrabies**
4 tablespoons **tomato paste**
1 tablespoon **virgin olive oil**
½ small **cucumber**, peeled, finely diced
6 **plum tomatoes**, finely diced
3 tablespoons **sesame seeds**, chopped

Peel the kohlrabies. Slice lengthwise. Whip together tomato paste and olive oil. Blend in remaining ingredients.

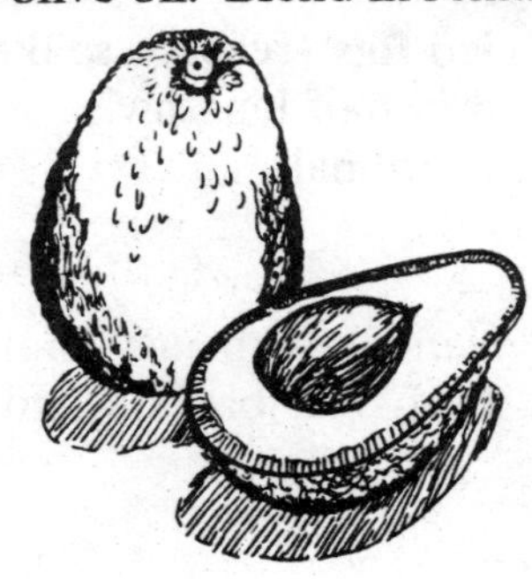

FRUIT DISHES

Apple Blueberry Pudding

1 cup organic **apple juice**
2 yellow-skinned **pears**, chopped
2 sweet **apples**, chopped
1 basket **blueberries**

Put apple juice in blender. Add pears and apples; puree. Fold in blueberries but don't blend. Scoop into dessert dishes.

Banana Blueberry Dish

Basket of **blueberries**
2 medium bananas

Separate basket of blueberries in half. Slice bananas into dish. Puree half the blueberries in blender. Spoon other half over bananas.

Banana Delight

4 pre-soaked **dried figs** (reserve soaking water)
2 **bananas**, sliced in half lengthwise
1 **sapote**, sliced (optional)
6 **red cherries**

Place figs in blender with just enough of the soaking water to puree. Pour over banana and sapote. Top with cherries.

Serves Two

Breakfast Parfait

In stemmed glasses, layer sliced **strawberries**, **kiwi**, **pear** slices, **blackberries** (slice in half). Repeat layers, ending with strawberries. Place either blackberries or a slice of kiwi in center.

Cherimoya, Kiwi & Grapes

2 **cherimoyas** (also called Custard Apples)
2 **kiwis**
1 cup **seedless grapes** (any variety)

Cut cherimoya in quarters. Remove as many seeds as possible. Remove from skin in bite-sized pieces with a spoon. Peel, quarter, and slice kiwi. Mix together. Puree grapes. Pour over fruit.

Citrus Fruit Delight

1 **pink grapefruit**, cut in half, sectioned
1 large **orange**, peeled (pull sections off and cut in thirds)
1 large **kiwi**, peeled, quartered lengthwise, sliced
½ cup finely diced celery

Combine fruit. Sprinkle with celery. Serve immediately.

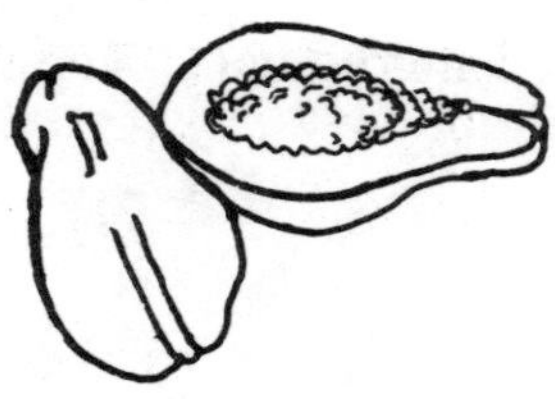

Serves Two

Feyoa Fruit Bowl

1 cup **gooseberries**
3 **feyoas** (also called pineapple guavas), peeled and cubed
1 **pear**, cubed
1 **kiwi**, peeled, cubed

Put half of gooseberries in blender and puree. Combine fruit and pour juice over top.

Morning Fruit Dish

3-4 **bananas**, sliced
1 **papaya**
1 small **mango**

Cut papaya in half. Remove seeds. Scoop out bite-sized pieces. Peel mango, cut pulp away from pit, and chop. Puree half and pour over fruit.

Pineapple & Kumquat

1½ cups **pineapple**, cut into chunks
¾ cup **kumquats**, seeded and sliced (keep skin on)
2 **kiwis**, peeled, quartered, sliced
¼ cup diced, tender center **celery**
6 **strawberries** (optional)

Combine first 5 ingredients. Top with strawberries.

Serves Two

Pear & Cherry with Plum Syrup

2 **pears**
1 cup fresh **cherries**, pitted
2 **plums**
½ cup pre-soaked **raisins** (reserve soaking water)

Quarter pears, remove seeds, and chop. Mix with cherries. Put plums and raisins in blender with just enough soaking water to blend. Pour over top.

Fruit Dish with Dried Apricot Topping

2 ripe **peaches**, peeled, cut into chunks
2 ripe **plums**, peeled, cut into chunks
6 **dried apricots** (pre-soak overnight; reserve soaking water)
½ cup **grapes**

Blend apricots and grapes with just enough soaking water to puree. Pour over peaches and plums.

Pear Apple Fruit Dish

2 **pears**
2 **apples**
1 cup **alfalfa sprouts**
½ cup pre-soaked **raisins** (or grapes or cherries)
⅔ cup unfiltered **apple juice**

Quarter pears and apples; remove seeds. Chop. Sprinkle sprouts on top. Garnish with raisins (or grapes or cherries). Pour juice over top.

Serves Two

FRUIT DRINKS

Apple Sapote Cherry Drink

2 cups organic **apple** juice
1 cup chopped **sapote**
½ cup **cherries**

Combine all ingredients in electric blender.

Banana Shake

1 small **papaya**, peeled, pitted, chopped
3 large pitted **dates**
2 ripe **bananas**, cut in quarters

Put papaya and dates in blender and puree. Put in banana and blend for five seconds. Scoop into dessert dishes.

Blueberry Apple Drink

2 cups organic **apple juice**
1 cup **blueberries**
1 cup white seedless **grapes**

Blend all ingredients in electric blender.

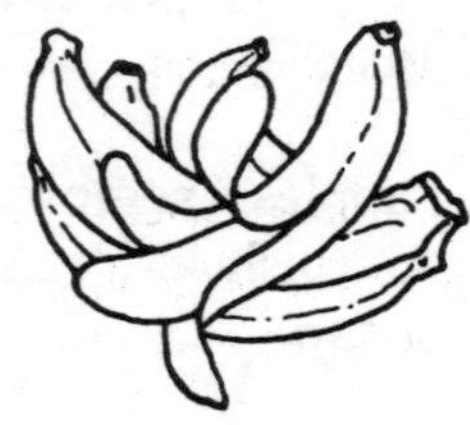

Serves Two

Cherry Apple Drink

1 cup fresh **cherries**, pitted
3 yellow **apples**, chopped (don't peel if skins aren't waxed)

Put cherries and apples in blender and liquefy.

Grape Apricot Drink

3 cups **grapes**
1 cup chopped **apricots**

Liquefy all ingredients in electric blender.

Orange Loganberry Drink

2 cups **orange juice**
1 cup **loganberries**
1 **celery stalk**, chopped

Liquefy all ingredients in electric blender.

Persimmon Shake

2 *ripe* **persimmons**, quartered
4 pre-soaked **dried figs**, quartered
2 pre-soaked **dried apricots**, quartered

Put all in blender and puree. Serve immediately.

Serves Two

PINEAPPLE DRINK

3 cups **pineapple chunks**
1 rib **celery***
1 **pear**, quartered, seeded
1 cup white seedless **grapes**

Combine all ingredients in blender and liquefy. Serve immediately.

*Celery is an alkaline vegetable. It neutralizes the acid in the pineapple.

APPLEBERRY DRINK

3 cups freshly made **apple juice**
1 cup **boysenberries**
1 cup **blackberries**

Put all in blender and liquefy.

PEACH, PEAR & PLUM DRINK

2 large **peaches**, quartered
2 large **plums**, quartered
2 **pears**, quartered
⅓ cup **blackberries**, mashed with fork

Combine peaches, plums, and pears in blender and liquefy. Pour into chilled juice glasses. Spoon blackberries over top.

SERVES TWO

FRUIT SYRUPS

Apricot-Fig Syrup

½ cup pre-soaked **dried apricots**
⅓ cup pre-soaked **dried figs** (reserve soaking water)

Soak dried apricots and figs overnight in just enough distilled water to cover.

Blend in an electric blender with just enough soaking water to puree. Pour over sweet or low-acid fruits.

Blueberry Apricot Syrup

½ cup **blueberries**
½ cup pre-soaked, chopped **dried apricots** (reserve soaking water)

Use just enough of the soaking water to puree in an electric blender. Pour over sweet or low-acid fruits.

Grape Plum Syrup

1 cup seedless **grapes**
1 large **plum**, pitted, quartered

Combine grapes and plum in blender or nut chopper. Puree. Pour over low-acid fruit dishes.

Date Apple Syrup

6 **dates**, pitted
½ cup **dried apples**
¾ cup seedless **sweet grapes**

Soak dates and apples in distilled water overnight (just enough to cover). Reserve soaking water.

Put grapes in blender and blend 5 seconds. Add dates and apples. Blend. Add only enough soaking water to give you the consistency you desire. Use over sweet or low-acid fruits.

Pineapple Syrup

2 **dried pineapples**
Distilled water

Put dried pineapples in a wide-mouth jar. Add enough distilled water to cover. Soak overnight.

Put pineapple and water in blender; blend to a creamy consistency. Add more distilled water if necessary.

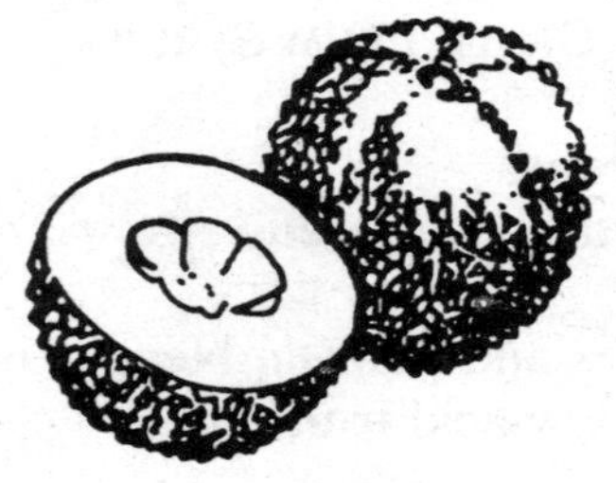

NUT AND SEED MILKS AND NUT BUTTERS

Nut and seed milks are highly nutritious, being high in protein and essential minerals such as calcium. They are easy to digest and simple to make.

When blending seeds or nuts, start by putting ½ cup of the given amount of water and all the seeds, meal, or nuts into a covered blender. Start with a low speed and increase to high. As the mixture thickens, add more water. Repeat until all the liquid is used up. Add more water if you desire a thinner consistency.

Use any one of the following: 1½ cups **almonds, cashews, sesame seeds, sunflower seeds**, or **pumpkin seeds**. Use 4 cups of **cold distilled water**.

When using almonds, it's best to soak them overnight and remove the bitter skins by blanching them with boiling water. The skins will be ready to squeeze off in less than a minute.

A nut butter can be made out of any kind of seed or nut (or combination of them). Use a nut chopper or a seed-nut mill, and grind only enough to use. Once the germ is exposed to the air, not only will it begin to oxidize (as all things in nature do), but it will soon lose some of its nutrients.

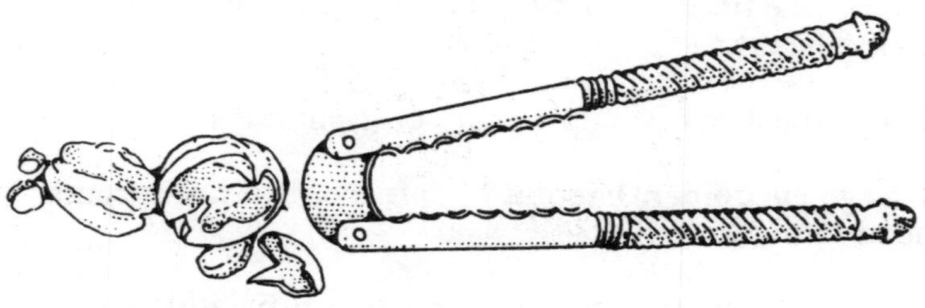

VEGETABLE DRINKS

Use only fresh, ripe vegetables, preferably organically grown. If regular supermarket-quality produce is used, it should be carefully washed. (See "How to Clean Vegetables" in Instructions for Recipes.)

Make only the amount of juice that will be used immediately. In storage, even under refrigeration, raw juices oxidize rapidly and lose their medicinal value after ten minutes.

Drink vegetable or fruit juices between meals or one hour before meals, but never with meals.

Combine the following groups in juicer:

2 or 3 **tomatoes**, 1 **celery** stalk, 1 small **cucumber**. (If not organic, remove skin.)

2 or 3 **beets**, 1 **celery** stalk, 1 small **cucumber**, 1 cup sliced **cabbage**.

Head lettuce, **carrots**, **string beans**, **bell peppers**.

2 or 3 **tomatoes**, 1 **celery** stalk, **yellow bell pepper**.

4 fresh **carrots** and tops, 1 small **jicama**, 1 **tomatillo**.

1 large **cucumber**, 1 large **beet**, 1 cup **sprouts**, handful of **string beans**.

2 or 3 **tomatoes**, ½ cup **corn**, 1 or 2 **parsnips**.

1 large **cucumber**, handful of **spinach**, handful **sprouts**, ¼ head lettuce.

¼ cup of sprouted **sunflower seeds** can be added to each group for a creamy drink.

SOUPS

Avocado Soup

2 Haas **avocados**, one divided in half
1 medium **cucumber**, **¾** chopped, ¼ diced small
2 large, ripe **tomatoes**, quartered
¼ cup chopped **watercress**

Remove avocado pulp with a tablespoon. Put 1½ of the avocados in blender with tomatoes and chopped **¾** cucumber. Blend until smooth. Pour into bowls. Stir in the remaining ½ avocado and diced ¼ cucumber. Garnish with watercress.

Creamy Avocado & Tomato Soup

2 cups **tomato juice** (made from fresh tomatoes in blender)
1 medium small **tomatillo**, chopped
1 heaping tablespoon **almond butter**
1 ripe Haas **avocado**

Remove avocado pulp with a tablespoon. Combine all ingredients in an electric blender in order given. Blend until smooth.

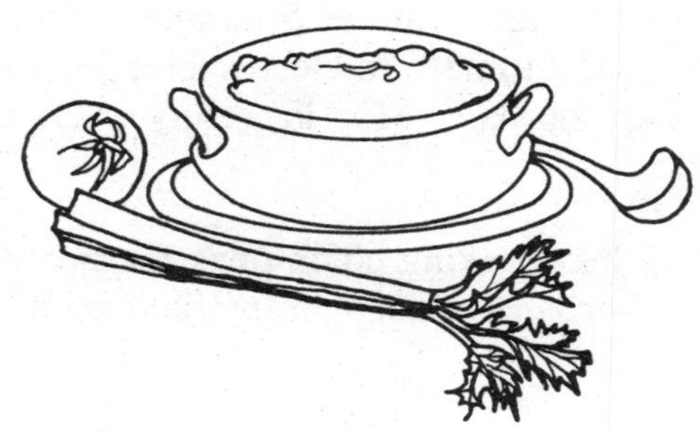

Serves Two

BARLEY CARROT SOUP*

¾ cup **barley**
1 cup **distilled water**
2 cups **carrot juice**
½ cup chopped **celery**
½ cup chopped **parsley**

Soak barley overnight in distilled water. Refrigerate.

When preparing meal, rinse barley. Cover with distilled water and simmer 5 minutes. Drain. Combine all ingredients.

*This dish requires soaking barley overnight.

CHICK PEA & TOMATO SOUP*

⅓ cup **dried chick peas** (they will swell to 3 times their size)
1½ cups **distilled water**
2 cups **tomato juice** (made in blender from fresh tomatoes)
½ cup diced **celery**
Watercress for garnish

When preparing meal, rinse chick peas. Drain. Cover with distilled water and simmer 5 minutes. Drain. Combine chick peas and tomato in electric blender and liquefy. Pour into soup bowls. Mix in celery. Garnish with watercress.

*This dish requires soaking chick peas for two days. See "How to Soak Garbanzo Beans" in Instructions for Recipes.

SERVES TWO

Corn Chowder

1-1½ cups **distilled water**
1 rib **celery**, chopped in 1" lengths
½ cup finely diced, tender rib of **celery**
1 cup shredded **jicama**
2 medium **parsnips**, peeled, shredded
2 ears **corn**, kerneled (set one aside)
4 **walnuts**, chopped
¼ cup minced **parsley**

Place half the amount of celery, jicama, parsnip, and corn in electric blender with just enough water to blend. Pour into large bowl. Blend other half. Pour in bowl. Mix in other ear of corn and diced celery.

Ladle into individual bowls. Garnish with walnuts and parsley.

Creamy Carrot & Avocado Soup

3 cups fresh **carrot juice**
1 large Haas **avocado**
Handful **alfalfa sprouts**, cut in thirds
Small sprig **parsley** or **cilantro**

Cut avocado in half. Place carrot juice and ½ avocado in blender. Blend until smooth.

Pour into individual soup bowls. Dice other half of avocado and add to soup. Add sprouts and parsley.

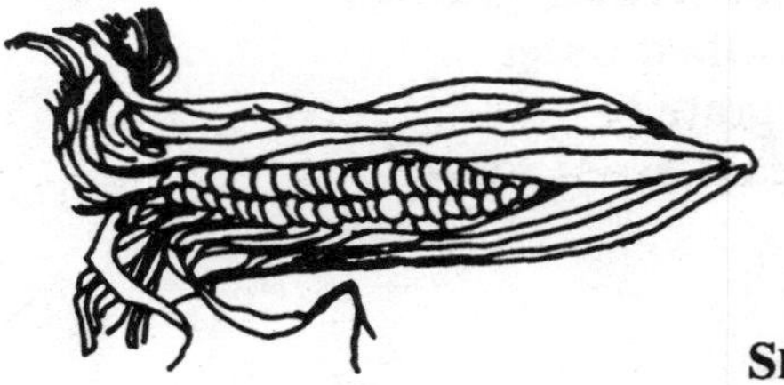

Serves Two

Cream of Tomato Soup

3 cups pureed **tomatoes** (with skins)
2 tablespoons **almond butter**
2 medium-small **plum tomatoes**, diced
½ cup **sunflower sprout tops**
(use bottoms for a salad)

Put pureed tomatoes (not plum tomatoes) and almond butter in blender. Puree. Pour into soup bowls. Sprinkle with plum tomatoes and sprouts.

Cream of Spinach Soup

3 cups chopped fresh **spinach**
1½ cups chopped **zucchini**
1½ cups warm **distilled water**
1 teaspoon **butter** or **virgin olive oil** (optional)
1 ear **corn**, kerneled

Blend spinach and zucchini. Melt butter in pot. Add soup and warm on low heat 2 minutes. Ladle into bowls. Sprinkle with corn.

Green Pea Soup

1 large Haas **avocado**, chopped
1½ cups **peas**
1 medium **zucchini**, grated
1¼ cups **distilled water**
1 **carrot**, grated
2 sprigs **parsley**, chopped

Serves Two

Blend avocado, peas, zucchini and water (use more if necessary) in blender until creamy. Mix in carrots. Garnish with parsley.

Life Force Soup

4 large **carrots**, grated
1 cup grated **jicama**
1 cup **parsley**
½ bunch **spinach**
2 large **tomatoes**, quartered
1 cup **alfalfa sprouts**

Puree all ingredients in electric blender until smooth.

Raw Borscht

4 small young **beets**
¼ medium head **cabbage**, sliced and chopped
1 cup **carrot juice**, made fresh in juicer
1 small *fresh* **jicama**, chopped in 1" squares
1 rib **celery**, chopped
1-1½ cups **distilled water**

Liquefy first 5 vegetables a bit at a time, using water as necessary, in electric blender. Pour into large bowl to mix. Ladle into individual bowls.

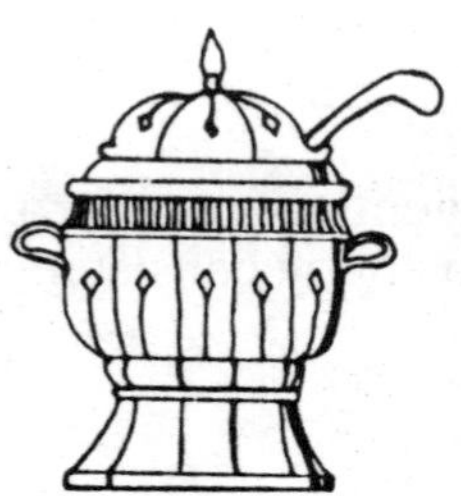

Serves Two

TOMATO VEGETABLE SOUP

3 cups freshly made **tomato juice**
1 ear **corn**, kerneled
¾ cup **peas**
½ cup diced **celery**
⅓ cup **watercress**
4 **walnuts**, chopped

Mix ingredients in large bowl. Ladle into individual soup bowls. Garnish with nuts and watercress.

COOL TOMATO SOUP

2 cups freshly made **tomato juice**
1½ medium **cucumbers**, peeled, chopped
½ medium **cucumber**, peeled, diced (set aside)
1 cup **alfalfa sprouts**, cut in thirds
1 small **yellow bell pepper**, finely diced
¼ cup **watercress** or **parsley**, chopped

Puree tomatoes and chopped cucumbers. Pour mixture into large bowl. Add next 4 ingredients. Ladle into individual bowls.

ZUCCHINI & PEA SOUP

3 medium **zucchini**, grated (about 3-3½ cups)
2 cups **peas**
1-1½ cups **distilled water**
½ cup diced **celery**
sprig of **parsley**

Blend first 4 ingredients in blender until smooth. Use only enough water for a soupy consistency. Pour into soup bowls. Mix in celery.

SERVES TWO

SALAD DRESSINGS

Note: don't put nut dressings on starchy vegetables.

Avocado-Carrot Dressing

1 cup **carrot juice**
1 small **avocado**, chopped
¼ cup **sesame seeds**

Put ingredients in blender. Blend until smooth.

Avocado-Corn Dressing

Juice of half a **pink grapefruit**
1 large ear sweet **corn**, kerneled
1 small **avocado**, chopped

Put juice from grapefruit in blender. Scrape "cream" from corn cob with a paring knife into a bowl. Add kernels and cream to blender. Add avocado. Liquefy until creamy.

Avocado & Cucumber Dressing

1 medium **cucumber**, peeled, chopped
1 small **avocado**, chopped
1 small **tomatillo**, quartered

Put cucumber in blender. Add tomatillo and liquefy. Add avocado. Liquefy until creamy.

CARROT-ALMOND DRESSING

1 cup **carrot juice**
4 ounces **almond butter**

Blend ingredients until smooth.

CREAMY CARROT DRESSING

½ cup **carrot juice**
1 rib **celery**, juiced
1 small **avocado**, chopped

Put ingredients in blender. Liquefy until creamy.

CREAMY CELERY DRESSING

¾ cup **distilled water**
2 ribs **celery**, chopped
1 small **zucchini**, unpeeled, chopped
¼ cup chopped **walnuts** or **almonds**
(remove almond skins by blanching)

Place all in blender. Liquefy until smooth.

TOMATO-TOMATILLO DRESSING

2 medium **tomatoes**, quartered
1 small **tomatillo**, chopped
½ cup chopped **celery**

Combine all in blender. Blend until smooth.

Tomato-Walnut Dressing

2 medium **tomatoes**, quartered
½ cup **walnuts**

Combine ingredients in blender and blend until creamy.

Tomatillo-Cucumber Dressing

1 medium **cucumber**, peeled, chopped
1 small **tomatillo**, chopped
2 tablespoons **Bragg's Liquid Aminos**

Put ingredients in blender and liquefy.

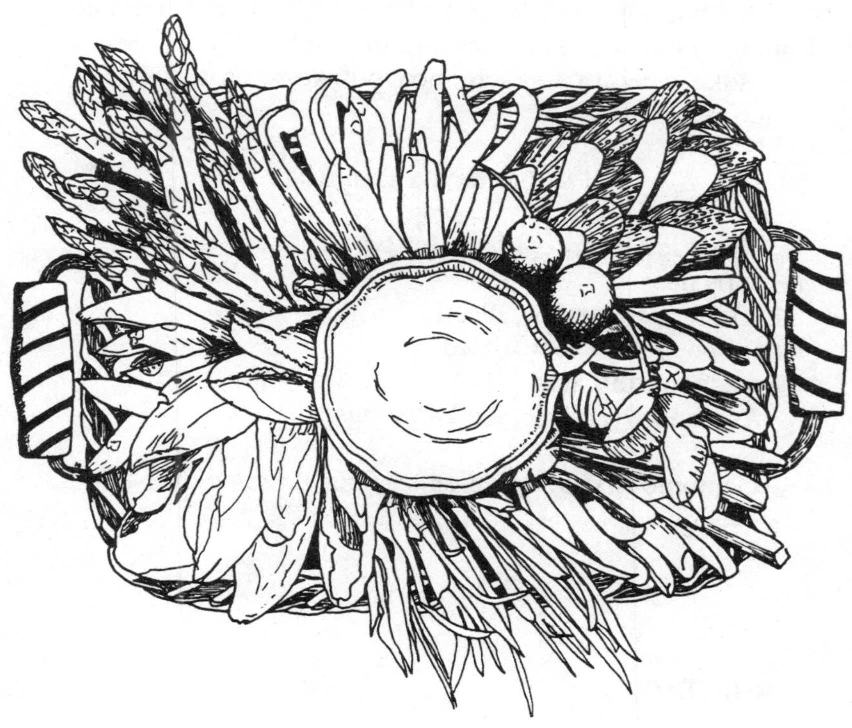

MAIN DISHES

JICAMA SALAD

1 medium **jicama**, cut in small cubes
2 medium **carrots**, grated
1 tender stalk **celery**, diced
½ cup **peas**
¼ teaspoon **cumin seed**
2 tablespoons **Bragg's Liquid Aminos**
1 medium **cucumber**, peeled, chopped
1 small **tomatillo**, chopped
1 small bunch **spinach**, stems removed, chopped

Combine jicama, carrots, celery, peas (if using frozen, just defrost) and cumin seed.

Put aminos, cucumber and tomatillo in blender and liquefy. Pour on vegetables and mix well.

Make a bed of spinach. Scoop mixture on top.

PEAS & SAVOY CABBAGE

Shredded **savoy cabbage** for two
1½ cups **peas**
1 medium **cucumber**, diced
1 **yellow bell pepper**, diced
½-1 teaspoon **dill seed**
Avocado Dressing (see Dressings)

Combine first 5 ingredients. Pour dressing over top.

SERVES TWO

Red Cabbage & Corn (I)

Red cabbage for two, shredded
2 cups **sunflower sprouts**
1 **cucumber**, sliced
1 ear **corn**, kerneled
½ teaspoon **caraway seed**
Tomatillo-Cucumber Dressing (see Dressings)

Mix cabbage and sprouts. Spread on plate leaving 1" around the edge. Sprinkle on caraway.

Place cucumber slices around the outer edge of plate. Spoon the corn in a circle next to cucumbers. Pour dressing over top.

Spinach & Jerusalem Artichoke

Spinach for two
1 cup sliced **Jerusalem artichokes**
(also known as sun chokes)
1 **red pepper**, diced
1 **yellow pepper**, diced
Tomatillo-Cucumber Dressing (see Dressings)

Break spinach into bite-sized pieces. Scrub artichokes well. Combine first four ingredients. Pour dressing over top.

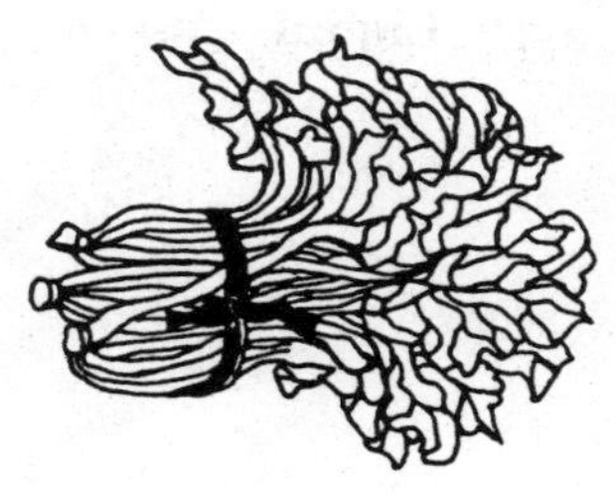

Serves Two

"SPAGHETTI, TOMATO SAUCE & CHEESE"

Grated **spaghetti squash** for two
¾ pound ripe **tomatoes**, quartered
Fresh **parsley** and **sweet basil**, minced
½ cup pre-soaked **garbanzo beans***
Distilled water

Rinse garbanzo beans. Put in small saucepan. Cover with distilled water. Simmer 5 minutes.

In the meantime, cut squash in half at the center. Refrigerate half for other use. Slice other half in thirds. Cut slices in half. Remove seeds. Slice off skin. Grate in a food processor.

Liquefy tomatoes in blender. Drain garbanzo beans. Grate. Put squash on plate. Pour tomato over it. Sprinkle on parsley and sweet basil. Sprinkle garbanzo "cheese" on top. Serve with a small green salad or on a bed of spinach.

*This recipe requires soaking garbanzos for two days. See "How to Soak Garbanzo Beans" in Instructions for Recipes.

SPAGHETTI SQUASH & AVOCADO

1 medium/small **spaghetti squash**
1 large **avocado**
2 medium **carrots**
2 tablespoons **Bragg's Liquid Aminos**
Spinach

SERVES TWO

Cut squash in half. Scoop out seeds from one half. Seal tightly with plastic wrap and refrigerate. Cut other half in 3 slices. Cut slices in half. Scrape out seeds with knife. Slice skins off. Set aside.

Scrub carrots well and grate coarsely. Grate squash. Cut avocado in half. Put liquid aminos in blender. Scoop half of avocado pulp into blender. Blend.

Mix squash and carrot. Scoop onto bed of spinach. Pour avocado dressing over top. Scoop out bite-sized portions of the other half of the avocado and place around the top.

STUFFED TOMATOES

4 medium **tomatoes**
½ cup **peas**
1 small **zucchini**, grated
1 ear of **corn**, kerneled
1 Haas **avocado**
2 tablespoons **Bragg's Liquid Aminos**
Boston lettuce

Cut stems from tomatoes. Cut in eighths not quite to the bottom. Refrigerate. Combine next three ingredients. Refrigerate.

Cut avocado in half. Remove pit. Cut thin slices in both directions while still in skin. Scoop pulp out with tablespoon. Put avocado and aminos in small bowl. Smash with fork. Blend refrigerated mixture into avocado.

Scoop mixture into center and spaces between tomato wedges. Place on bed of lettuce.

SERVES TWO

Vegetable Sushi

1 large ear **corn**
1 large **avocado**
¾ cup **red** and **yellow bell peppers**, diced
Sheets of **nori**

Kernel corn. Be sure to scrape the cream off the cob and keep it separate from the kernels.

Follow directions on nori package. Scoop avocado pulp into a small bowl. Add corn cream. Smash with fork. Mix in peppers. Scoop onto nori and roll.

Note: you can make extra for lunch at work.

Zucchini & Avocados with Carrots

Grated **zucchini** for two
1 large Haas **avocado**
1 large **carrot**, grated (to make 1 cup)
2 tablespoons **Bragg's Liquid Aminos**
½ teaspoon **dill seed** (optional)
4 large **Romaine** leaves, sliced in thin strips

Grate zucchini and carrot with a coarse grater. Cut avocado in half. Remove pit. Cut thin slices in both directions while still in skin. Remove with a tablespoon into bowl with zucchini and carrot. Sprinkle with soy and dill. Mix. Make a bed of greens with lettuce. Scoop mixture on top.

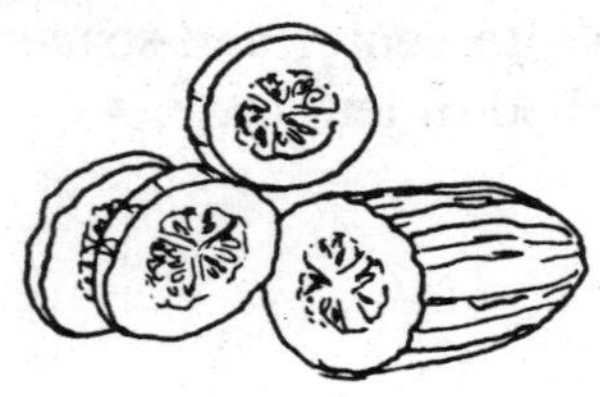

Serves Two

Yam & Spinach Patties

¾ cup **oatmeal**
½ cup **distilled water**
1 bunch **spinach**, stems removed, chopped
2 cups grated **yams**
¼ cup finely diced **celery**
½ cup chopped **walnuts**
1 ear **corn**, kerneled
2 tablespoons **virgin olive oil**
Handful **snow peas**, stems and strings removed
2 pats **butter**

Soak oatmeal 5 minutes. Mix occasionally with a fork. Oatmeal should not be watery.

Steam yams and celery 3 minutes. Add spinach and let stand one more minute. Transfer to a covered bowl.

Put snow peas in steamer and steam 3 minutes. While they are steaming, combine oatmeal, spinach, yams, celery, walnuts, and corn. Include the "cream" scraped from the cob. Form into patties.

Heat oil in skillet. Sauté patties 2 minutes on each side. Serve with buttered snow peas on the side.

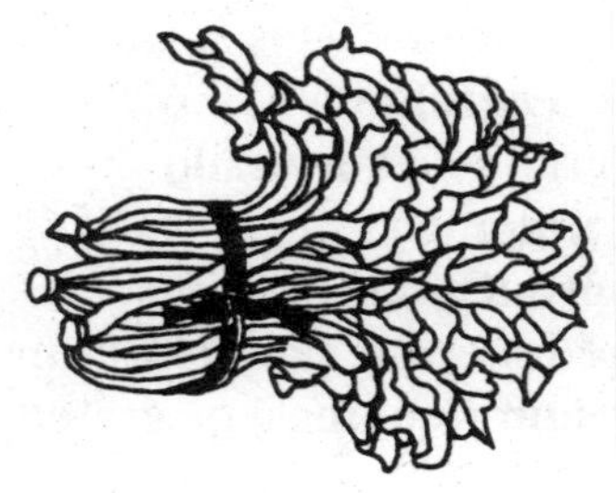

Serves Two

TRANSITION RECIPES
(partly steamed, with raw ingredients)

Soups and Stews

ASPARAGUS SOUP

1 cup **distilled water**
Asparagus for two, sliced in 1" pieces
(set aside tips)
1 cup grated **jicama**
1 stalk **celery**, cut in 1" lengths
½ cup **celery**, finely diced
⅓ cup **watercress**, chopped
½ cup **walnuts**, chopped

Use distilled water to steam asparagus 4 minutes. Use same water to liquefy jicama and celery in blender (add more water as necessary). Add asparagus and blend again. Transfer to large bowl. Mix in watercress.

Pour into individual bowls. Garnish with asparagus tips and walnuts.

AVOCADO & CAULIFLOWER SOUP

3 cups chopped **cauliflower**
1 medium to large Haas **avocado**
1 cup distilled **water**
1 cup **alfalfa sprouts**, cut in thirds
Choice of the following garnishes: **peas**,
corn, diced **plum tomatoes**, or grated **carrot**.

SERVES TWO

Steam cauliflower 5 minutes with distilled water. Remove from heat and keep in covered bowl.

Seed avocado, and cut thin slices in both directions while still in skin. Remove pulp from skin. Place both in blender with steaming water. Add more water as necessary. Blend until smooth.

Pour into soup dishes. Add sprouts. Garnish.

Broccoli Zucchini Soup

Broccoli for two
2 cups chopped **zucchini**
1 cup **distilled water**
½ cup finely diced **celery**
½ small **red pepper**, diced
⅓ cup **pignolias (pine nuts)**

Cut broccoli into florets. Steam 4 minutes.

Blend broccoli, zucchini, and steaming water in blender until smooth. Add more water as necessary.

Pour into soup dishes. Mix in celery, pepper, and pine nuts.

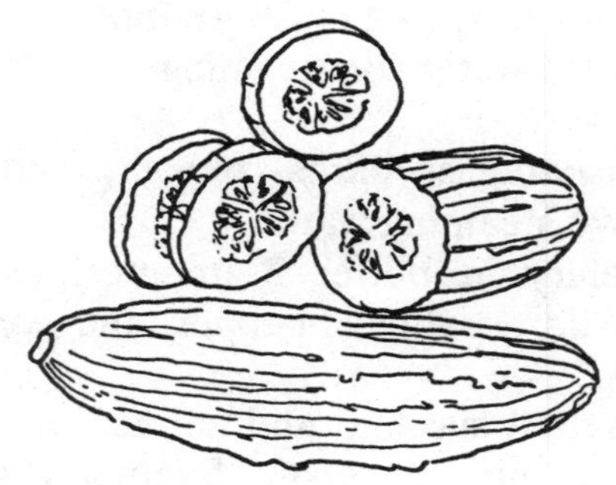

Serves Two

CAULIFLOWER & CORN SOUP

Chopped **cauliflower** for two
1¼ cups **distilled water**
1 medium grated **parsnip**
1 ear of **corn**, kerneled
¼ cup chopped **watercress**

Steam cauliflower 5 minutes.

Puree cauliflower, parsnip, and steaming water in blender until smooth. Add more water as necessary. Add corn, but don't blend. Mix with wooden spoon.

Pour into bowls. Garnish with watercress.

ASPARAGUS STEW

Asparagus for two, cut in 1¼" lengths
4 **okras**, sliced
1 small **red bell pepper**, chopped
2-3 **bok choy** stems, cut down center, sliced thin
¼ cup diced **celery**
3 pats **butter** or 1 tablespoon **virgin olive oil**
1 medium, unpeeled **zucchini**, liquefied in blender
2 tablespoons **Bragg's Liquid Aminos**
1 cup **distilled water** for steaming

Steam asparagus, okras, pepper, and bok choy 4 minutes. Save steaming water.

Sauté celery in butter 3 minutes, using a 3-quart saucepan. Add asparagus, pepper, and bok choy. Sauté for 1 minute.

Add liquefied zucchini and aminos to steaming water and heat. Pour into saucepan. Simmer 1 minute.

SERVES TWO

Asparagus, Parsnip & Carrot

¾ pound **asparagus**, cut in 1" pieces (set tops aside)
1 large **parsnip**, peeled, grated
1 medium **carrot**, peeled, grated
3 pats **butter** or 2 tablespoons **virgin olive oil**

Steam asparagus bottoms 4 minutes. Heat butter in a 10" skillet on medium heat. Add all vegetables and sauté 3 minutes. Keep covered. Turn with spatula several times.

Beets, Cauliflower & Okras

4 small **beets**, julienned
2 cups **cauliflower** florets
3 large **okras**, sliced
3 pats **butter**
2 tablespoons **Bragg's Liquid Aminos**
½ tablespoon **caraway seed**

Steam vegetables 6 minutes. Remove steamer. Put pot cover on vegetables to keep warm. Discard steaming water.

Melt butter in pot. Add aminos and caraway seeds. Heat. Add vegetables and mix well.

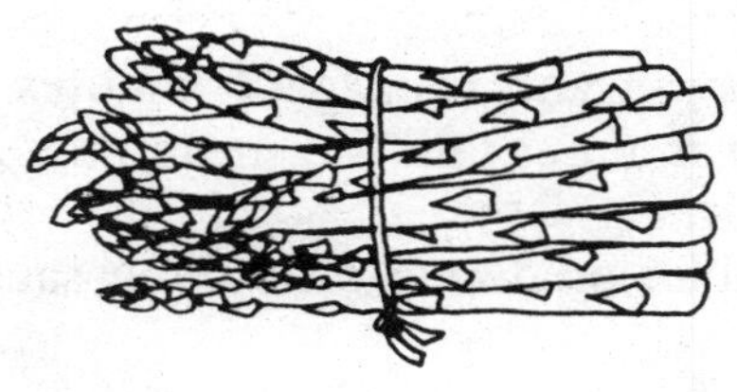

Serves Two

BEETS, BARLEY & PEAS*

1 cup uncooked **barley**
2 cups **distilled water**
2 medium **beets**, grated
¾ cup **peas**
3 pats **butter**
2 tablespoons **Bragg's Liquid Aminos**
Sunflower sprouts

Soak barley overnight in distilled water. When preparing meal, drain and rinse well.

Steam beets 5 minutes. Add peas. Steam 1 minute longer. Remove steamer and vegetables from pot; keep covered with pot top. Discard steaming water.

Put aminos in saucepan. Add butter and melt. Add vegetables and mix.

*This dish requires overnight soaking of barley.

BROCCOLI, SAVOY CABBAGE & CARROTS

1 head **broccoli**, cut into florets
3 cups sliced **savoy cabbage**
1 large **carrot**, sliced diagonally
½ can **cream of celery soup**
¼ cup **distilled water**
¼ cup chopped **walnuts** (optional)

Steam broccoli and cabbage 4 minutes. Add carrot. Steam 2 more minutes. In the meantime, combine soup and water; heat.

Put vegetables on dinner dish. Pour sauce over top.

SERVES TWO

Brussels Sprouts, Rutabaga & Carrots

1 medium-small **rutabaga**, grated
6 medium **Brussels sprouts**, sliced thin
1 medium **carrot**, grated
½ can **cream of celery soup**
3 pats **butter**
1 cup **distilled water** for steaming

Steam rutabaga 3 minutes. Add Brussels sprouts and steam 3 minutes longer. Add carrot and steam an additional 2 minutes.

Remove steamer. Measure ½ cup steaming water; combine with soup and butter. Heat. Add vegetables and mix.

Butternut Squash Patties

1 small **butternut squash**
⅓ cup ground **almonds**
⅓ cup ground **sunflower seeds**
¼ cup finely diced **celery**
⅓ cup minced **parsley**
2 tablespoons **virgin olive oil**

Wash and cut squash 2" thick. Slice peel off. Remove seeds. Grate.

Steam squash 3 minutes. Combine with remaining ingredients. Mix well and form into patties.

Heat oil in a 10" skillet. Sauté patties 2 minutes on each side. Serve with a green vegetable.

Serves Two

Cabbage & Two-Pepper Casserole

4 cups shredded **cabbage**
1 small **red bell pepper**
1 small **yellow bell pepper**
2 tablespoons **virgin olive oil**
1 teaspoon **caraway seed**

Remove pulp and seeds from peppers; slice. Steam peppers and cabbage 5 minutes.

Heat oil in a 10" skillet. Sauté cabbage and peppers 4 minutes. Sprinkle with caraway seed.

Carrots, Kale & Mushrooms

4 medium **carrots**, sliced thin
1 small bunch **kale**, chopped
1 cup sliced **mushrooms**
1 medium **zucchini**, grated
3 pats **butter**
2 tablespoons **Bragg's Liquid Aminos**

Steam carrots, kale, and mushrooms 4 minutes. Add zucchini and steam 1 minute longer. Remove steamer and vegetables from pot; keep covered. Discard water.

Put aminos in saucepan. Add butter and melt. Add vegetables and mix.

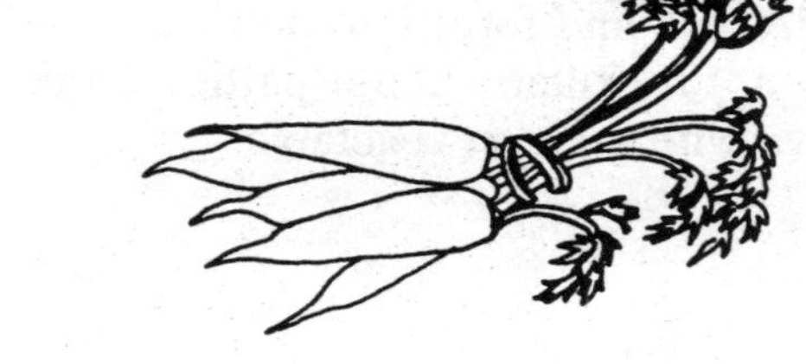

Serves Two

CAULIFLOWER, SNOW PEAS & CORN

1 small head **cauliflower**, cut into florets
1 cup **snow peas**, cut in half
1 ear **corn**, kerneled
2 handfuls **sunflower sprouts**
2 sprigs **parsley**, minced
2 tablespoons **Bragg's Liquid Aminos**

Steam cauliflower 5 minutes. Add snow peas and steam 2 more minutes.

Place steamed vegetables in bowl; mix in corn. Make a bed of sprouts and scoop mixture on top.

CARROT & SPINACH CRUNCH

2 large **carrots**, sliced thin diagonally
1 medium **parsnip**, sliced thin diagonally
1 bunch **spinach**, stems removed, chopped
2 pats **butter** (room temperature)
2 tablespoons **Bragg's Liquid Aminos**

Steam carrots and parsnips 5 minutes. Add spinach and steam 1 minute longer.

Put butter in a bowl. Add carrots and spinach. Mix. Sprinkle with aminos.

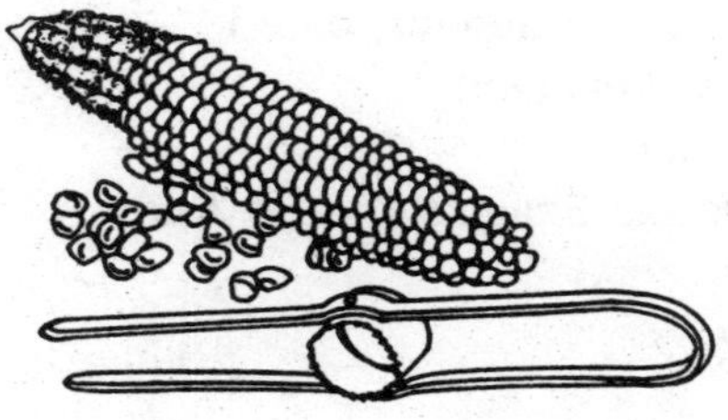

SERVES TWO

CAULIFLOWER, AVOCADO & CORN

1 small head **cauliflower**, cut into florets
1 ear **corn**, kerneled
1 medium **carrot**, grated
1 medium **cucumber**, peeled, chopped
1 small **tomatillo**, chopped
2 tablespoons **Bragg's Liquid Aminos**
1 small head **spinach**, stems removed, chopped
1 large Haas **avocado**

Steam cauliflower 7 minutes.

Put cucumber, tomatillo, and aminos in blender. Get a firm hold on top and bottom and gently shake the blender while it runs until the contents liquefy.

Prepare a bed of spinach. Cut avocado in half. Remove pit. Keep avocado in skin while cutting thin slices vertically and horizontally. Remove with tablespoon when ready to use.

Layer cauliflower, avocado, carrot, and corn over spinach. Pour cucumber dressing over top.

GREEN BEANS, CORN, MUSHROOMS & RED PEPPER

2 cups sliced **green beans**
1 cup sliced **mushrooms**
1 small **red bell pepper**, diced
1 ear **corn**, kerneled
2 pats **butter**
2 tablespoons **Bragg's Liquid Aminos**

SERVES TWO

Steam beans, mushrooms, and pepper 5 minutes. Add corn and steam 1 minute longer. Remove steamer and vegetables from pot. Discard water.

Put aminos in saucepan. Add butter and melt. Add cream scraped from corn cob. Add vegetables and mix.

GREEN BEAN, PARSNIP & OKRA CRUNCH

2 cups diagonally sliced **green beans**
4 **okras**, sliced
1 cup sliced **parsnip**
2 heaping tablespoonfuls **almond butter**
⅛-¼ cup **distilled water**
¼ cup slivered **almonds** (optional)

Steam vegetables 6 minutes. In the meantime, put almond butter in blender or nut chopper. Blend, gradually adding water until syrupy.

Place vegetables on plate. Pour almond butter over top. Garnish with slivered almonds.

KALE, PARSNIP & CARROT

1 bunch **kale**, scraped away from stem, chopped
1 medium **parsnip**, grated
1 medium **carrot**, grated
2 pats **butter**
2 tablespoons **Bragg's Liquid Aminos**

Steam first 3 ingredients 3 minutes. Remove steamer from pot. Discard water.

Heat aminos and butter until butter melts. Add vegetables and mix.

SERVES TWO

KALE, GARBANZO & PEPPERS*

½ cup dried **garbanzo beans**
2 cups **distilled water**
1 bunch **kale**, scraped from stem, chopped
1½ cups chopped **red** and **yellow bell peppers**
2 pats **butter**
2 tablespoons **Bragg's Liquid Aminos**

Soak garbanzo beans overnight. When preparing meal, rinse and drain well.

Steam garbanzo beans 5 minutes. Add kale and steam 2 minutes longer. Remove steamer from pot; discard water.

Heat aminos and butter until butter melts. Add vegetables. Mix.

PARSNIPS, CARROTS & CORN

2 cups sliced **parsnips**
1 cup grated **carrots**
1 **corn cob**, kerneled
Spinach

Peel parsnips. Steam 5 minutes. Add carrots. Steam 2 minutes.

Make a bed of spinach. Mix vegetables. Be sure to scrape "cream" off cob. Scoop onto a bed of spinach.

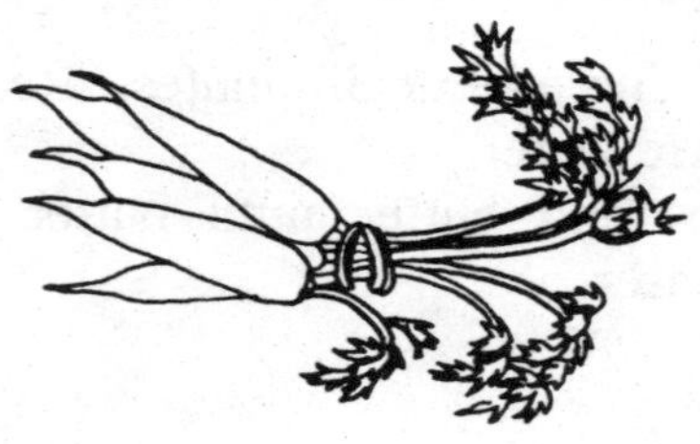

SERVES TWO

PASTA & SNOW PEAS

⅔ cup uncooked **elbow macaroni**
2 cups sliced **snow peas**
1 large **red bell pepper**, halved, seeded, sliced thin
2 pats **butter**
¼ cup diced **celery**
1 small **zucchini**, chopped
⅓ cup **distilled water**
1 *cup* chopped **parsley**

Cook macaroni according to package directions. While macaroni is cooking, steam snow peas and pepper 3 minutes.

Melt butter in 3-quart saucepan. Sauté celery. Liquefy zucchini with water in blender. Bring to simmer in saucepan. Add all ingredients. Simmer 30 seconds.

PASTA, BROCCOLI & WALNUTS

½ cup uncooked **elbow macaroni**
2 cups **broccoli** florets
1 rib **celery**, sliced diagonally
1 large **tomato**, chopped small
2 plum **tomatoes**, chopped small
½ cup chopped **walnuts**

Cook macaroni according to package directions. While macaroni is cooking, steam broccoli and celery 5 minutes.

Put tomatoes and walnuts in large bowl. Add broccoli and celery, and macaroni. Mix.

SERVES TWO

Peas & Rutabaga

1 small **rutabaga**, peeled, grated
1 cup **peas**
1 **red bell pepper**, diced
2 pats **butter**
2 tablespoons **Bragg's Liquid Aminos**
½ teaspoon **caraway**

Steam rutabaga 6 minutes. Add pepper and peas. Steam 1 minute longer. Remove steamer from pot. Keep vegetables covered. Discard water.

Heat aminos and butter until butter is melted. Add vegetables and mix.

Potato, Spinach & Okra Stew

2 medium **new potatoes**, peeled, cut in half, sliced ⅜" thick
6 large **okras**, sliced
1 bunch **spinach**, remove stems, chop
1 can **cream of potato soup**
½ cup **distilled water**

Steam potatoes and okras 5 minutes. Add spinach and steam 1 minute longer.

In the meantime, bring soup and water to simmer in saucepan. Use as sauce for vegetables.

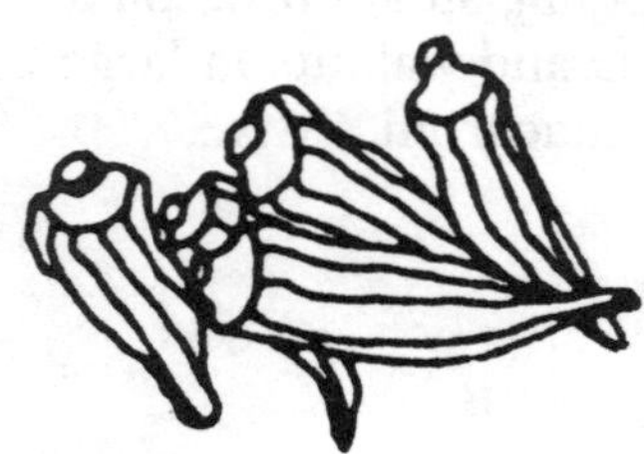

Serves Two

RED CABBAGE & CORN (II)

4 cups shredded **red cabbage**
1 cup sliced **Chinese peas** or **string beans**
1 ear **corn**, kerneled
2 tablespoons **Bragg's Liquid Aminos**
⅓ cup **distilled water**
1 medium **zucchini**, chopped

Steam cabbage and string beans 5 minutes. If using Chinese peas, steam the last 3 minutes.

Put aminos, water, and zucchini in blender. Add "cream" scraped from corn cob. Blend until creamy. Heat in saucepan.

Put vegetables in bowl. Add zucchini sauce. Mix and serve.

SAVOY CABBAGE, AVOCADO & PEAS

4 cups shredded **savoy cabbage**
2 medium Haas **avocados**
1 cup **peas**
2 tablespoons **Bragg's Liquid Aminos**
¼ cup **distilled water**
1 medium **zucchini**, chopped

Steam cabbage 4 minutes. Cut avocados in half. Remove pit. While still in skin, cut horizontally and vertically. Set aside.

Put aminos, zucchini, and the pulp of *one* avocado in blender. Blend until creamy.

Put cabbage and peas (if using frozen peas, just defrost) in bowl. Mix. Add chopped avocado. Mix gently.

Scoop on dinner dish. Pour dressing over top.

SERVES TWO

Potato Salad

5 to 7 small **red potatoes**, washed well
1 cup diced **red** and **yellow bell pepper**
⅓ cup diced **celery**
1 sprig **parsley**, minced
½ teaspoon **dill seed**
½ teaspoon **powdered kelp**
1 small **tomatillo**, minced
2 tablespoons **Bragg's Liquid Aminos**
1 medium **cucumber**
1 medium-small **tomatillo**, chopped

Put potatoes in pot. Cover with water. Bring to a boil. Simmer with cover on until barely done (about 5-8 minutes, depending on size).

Discard water. Cool off potatoes with running cold water. Fill pot with cold water and drain several times. Put potatoes in a covered casserole dish and refrigerate until cold.

When preparing meal, cut vegetables (small tomatillo only). Dice potatoes, add to vegetables, and Refrigerate.

Blend aminos, cucumber, and medium-small tomatillo until creamy. Pour over vegetables and mix.

Spaghetti Squash, Snow Peas & Tomatoes

½ medium **spaghetti squash**
1½ cups **distilled water**
1 *cup* chopped **parsley**
1 cup **snow peas**
2 medium **tomatoes**, chopped
4 **plum tomatoes**, chopped small

Serves Two

Cut squash into 2" slices. Slice skins off. Remove seeds. Grate. Steam 3 minutes.

Put 2 medium tomatoes in blender. Blend until smooth.

Remove squash from steamer into a 3-quart saucepan. Add parsley. Put heat on low to keep warm. Put snow peas in steamer 2 minutes.

Add tomato sauce and plum tomatoes to squash and mix. Turn heat to medium 1 minute.

Scoop mixture on dinner dishes. Place snow peas in a pinwheel design around dish.

SPINACH, BARLEY & BEETS

1 cup uncooked **barley***
1½ cups **distilled water**
2 medium-small **beets**, peeled, julienned
1 small bunch **spinach**, stems removed, chopped
2 pats **butter**
2 tablespoons **Bragg's Liquid Aminos**
½ teaspoon **dill seed**

Soak barley in distilled water overnight. When preparing meal, rinse barley and drain well.

Steam beets 5 minutes. Add spinach and steam 1 minute longer. Remove vegetables from steamer. Cover with pot top. Discard water.

Heat aminos and butter until butter melts. Put vegetables on dish. Pour sauce over top. Sprinkle with dill seed.

*Note: this recipe requires soaking of barley overnight.

SERVES TWO

Squash, Spinach & Corn

1 medium/small **butternut squash**
½ cup **celery**, sliced diagonally
2 pats **butter**
2 tablespoons **virgin olive oil**
1 ear **corn**, kerneled
1 bunch **spinach**, stems removed

Wash squash. Do not peel. Cut top of squash ¾" thick. Cut lower section, where seeds are, 1" thick. Scrape seeds out with a knife. Steam 7 minutes. Add celery. Steam 2 minutes longer.

Put butter and oil in skillet. Turn heat to medium. Add squash and celery. Sauté for 3 or 4 minutes. Keep covered.

Steam spinach 45 seconds. Combine all ingredients in skillet. Slice squash skin off when eating.

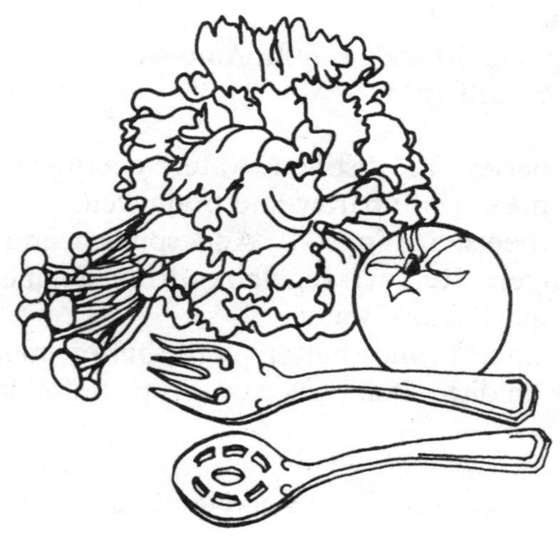

Serves Two

SPINACH, BRUSSELS SPROUTS & CORN

4-6 **Brussels sprouts**
1 ear **corn**, kerneled
1 large **carrot**, grated
½ bunch **spinach**
3 heaping tablespoons **almond butter**
⅓ cup **distilled water**

Steam Brussels sprouts 3 minutes. Add carrot. Steam 1 minute. Add spinach. Steam 1 minute longer.

Put water in blender or nut chopper. Add almond butter. Liquefy.

Put vegetables on plate. Pour sauce over top.

STUFFED PEPPERS WITH BARLEY*

2 large **yellow bell peppers**
¾ cup uncooked **barley**
½ cup **peas**
2 **plum tomatoes**, diced
2 large **tomatoes**, chopped
3 fresh **oregano leaves**, minced

Soak barley in 1½ cups distilled water overnight. When preparing meal, simmer 5 minutes. Drain.

Cut peppers from top to bottom. Remove seeds, but don't cut off stem. Combine barley with peas and plum tomato.

Puree regular tomatoes and oregano in blender. Add 6 tablespoons to barley mixture to moisten. Scoop mixture into peppers. Pour rest of dressing over peppers.

*Note: this recipe requires soaking barley overnight.

SERVES TWO

YAMS & SAVOY CABBAGE

2 cups grated **yams**
1 cup thinly sliced **savoy cabbage**
1 ear **corn**, kerneled
⅓ pound **snow peas**, stems and strings removed
3 heaping tablespoons **almond butter**
⅓ cup **distilled water**

Steam yams and cabbage 5 minutes. Combine with corn. Place snow peas on dish in a pinwheel design. Scoop yam mixture in center.

Put almond butter and water in blender. Liquefy. Pour over top.

YAM & WALNUT LOAF

¾ cup **oatmeal**
½ cup **distilled water**
2 cups grated **yams**
½ cup finely chopped **walnuts**
1 ear **corn**, kerneled
¼ cup minced **celery**
Salad greens

Pour water over oatmeal. Let stand 5 minutes. Steam yams 3 minutes.

Combine yams and oatmeal with walnuts, corn, and celery. Mix. Form into individual loaves. Place on salad greens.

SERVES TWO

BIBLIOGRAPHY

Main Sources

Correct Food Combining for Easy Digestion and Wonderful Health, prepared by T.C. Fry, Health Excellence Systems, 1108 Regal Row, Manchaca, TX 78652.

Food Combining Simplified, Dennis Nelson, P.O. Box 872-B, Santa Cruz, CA 95061. (Also see Recommended Reading.)

Health Reporter, 20 volumes, T.C. Fry et al., Health Excellence Systems (above).

Superior Nutrition, Dr. Herbert M. Shelton, Willow Publishing, Inc., San Antonio, TX 1987.

The Original Back to Eden, Jethro Kloss, Benedict Lust Publications, Box 404, New York, NY 10156.

What's Wrong with Eating Meat?, Vistara Parham, PCAP Publications, 97-38 42nd Avenue, Corona, NY 11368.

Secondary Sources

Be Your Own Doctor, Ann Wigmore, Hemisphere Press, New York.

Free Yourself from Digestive Pain: A Guide to Preventing and Curing Your Digestive Illness, J. Danzie, Prentice-Hall, Englewood Cliffs, NJ: 1984.

Gastrointestinal Disease: Pathophysiology Diagnosis Management, Marvin Sleisinger and John Fordtran, Saunders, Philadelphia, PA: 1983, 3rd Edition.

How to Get Along with Your Stomach: A Complete Guide for the Prevention and Treatment of Stomach Disorders, Nancy Nugent, Anchor-Doubleday, Garden City, NY: 1979.

Human Nutrition, Benjamin T. Burton, H.J. Heinz Co., 1976.

New Family Medical Guide, Edwin Kiester, Jr., Editor, Better Homes and Gardens Books: 1989.

Nutrition Against Disease, Roger J. Williams, Bantam Books, New York, 1973.

Nutrition and Diet Therapy, 3rd Edition, Sue Rodwell Williams, C.V. Mosby Co., St. Louis, 1977.

Prevention's New Encyclopedia of Common Diseases, by the editors of Prevention Magazine, Rodale Press, Emmaus, PA: 1984.

Physiology of the Digestive Tract, Horace Davenport, Year Book Medical: 1982.

The Great American Stomach Book: How Your Digestion Works and What to Do When It Doesn't, Maureen Mylander, Ticnor & Fields, New Haven, CT: 1982.

The Digestive System, Robert J. Bolt, John Wiley & Sons, Inc., 1983.

The American Medical Association: Encyclopedia of Medicine, Charles B. Clayman, M.D., Medical Editor, Random House, NY: 1989.

The Milk of Human Kindness Is Not Pasteurized, Dr. William Campbell Douglass, Last Laugh Publishers, 2250 Windy Hill Road, Suite 315, Marietta, GA 30067.

Understanding Nutrition, 2nd Edition, E.N. Whitney & E.M.M Hamilton, West Publishing Co., 1981.

RECOMMENDED READING

The Christ Diet
by Charles J. Hunt III
Heartquake Publishing
P.O. Box 593
La Jolla, CA 92038

Original Diet: Raw Vegetarian Guide and Recipe Book
by Karen Cross Whyte
Troubador Press
385 Fremont
San Francisco, CA 94105

Raw Energy
by Leslie and Susannah Kenton
Warner Books, Inc.
666 Fifth Avenue
New York, NY 10103

The Uncook Book:
Raw Food Adventures To A New Health High
by Elizabeth and Dr. Elton Baker
Communication Creativity
433 Fourth Street
P.0. Box 213
Saguache, CO 81149

Why Christians Get Sick
by Rev. George H. Malkmus
Hallelujah Acres Publishing
Eidson, Tennessee 37731

Fit for Life
by Harvey and Marilyn Diamond

A New Way of Eating
by Harvey & Marilyn Diamond

Living Health
by Harvey & Marilyn Diamond
Warner Books, Inc.
666 Fifth Avenue
New York, NY 10103

Your Heart Your Planet
by Harvey Diamond
Hay House, Inc.
501 Santa Monica Boulevard
Santa Monica, CA 90406

Light Eating for Survival
by Marcia Madhuri Acciardo
21st Century Publications
P.O. Box 702
Fairfield, IA 52556

Dick Gregory's Natural Diet for Folks Who Eat: Cookin' with Mother Nature
Perennial Library
Harper & Row, Publishers
New York

THE JUNK FOOD WITHDRAWAL MANUAL
by Monte Kline
Total Life Ministries
P.O. Box D
Eagle Point, OR 97524

Better Health with Foot Reflexology: The Original Ingham Method™
by Dwight C. Byers
Ingham Publishing, Inc.
Saint Petersburg, Florida

The Miracles of Rebound Exercise
The National Institute of Reboundology
& Health, Inc., 1979
Bothell, Washington

Blatant Raw Foodist Propaganda!
by Joe Alexander
Blue Dolphin Publishing, 1990
Grass Valley, California

Hand Reflexology: Key to Perfect Health
Mildred Carter
Parker Publishing Company, Inc.
West Nyack, NY 10994

Food Combining Simplified is available on a 60-minute tape for visually impaired people, or for commuters who like to learn while driving, etc. Send $5 to Dennis Nelson, P.O. Box 872-B, Santa Cruz, CA 95061. The book is available for $2.

Nelson also offers a biannual newsletter titled *Fruition*. It promotes public access fruit trees and community food-tree nurseries, as well as education for achieving superior health simply and naturally. Rates: $10/year. Sample issue $2.

RESOURCES

Raw Food Preparation Classes

Phyllis Avery's Raw Food Preparation Classes
Hygeia Publishing
1358 Fern Way
Vista, CA 92083

Sheila Gabayson, Owner/Operator
Garden Taste Restaurant
1555 Camino Del Mar
Del Mar, CA 92014
(619) 793-1500

Ann Wigmore Institute
(Workshops in raw food preparation.)
196 Commonwealth Avenue
Boston, MA 02116
(617) 267-9424

Sylvia Green Living Foods Workshops
Los Angeles, California
(310) 399-5612

The Optimum Health Institute
(A residential facility offering raw food preparation.)
6970 Central Avenue
Lemon Grove, CA 91945
(619) 464-3346

Kim Sproul and James Dina, roving teachers.
Contact Hygeia Press for their latest address.

Natural Hygiene Organizations

The American Natural Hygiene Society
P.O. Box 30630
Tampa, FL 33630
(818) 855-6607

The Canadian Natural Hygiene Society
Attn: Joe Aaron
P.O. Box 235, Station "T"
Toronto, ON M6B 4A1
Canada

GetWell * StayWell, America!
Attn: Victoria BidWell
1776 The Hygiene Joy Way
Mt. Vernon, WA 98273
(206) 428-3687
Write or call for a fun, free, fabulous, 150-page catalog!

Health Excellence Systems
Attn: T.C. Fry
1108 Regal Row
Manchaca, TX 78652
(512) 280-5566

Hygienic Community Network
2732 W. College Street
Springfield, MO 65802
(417) 831-3188

Natural Hygiene, Incorporated
Attn: Jo Willard
P.O. Box 2132
Huntington, CT 06084
(203) 929-1557

Orkos Institute
584 Castro Street
San Francisco, CA 94114

The Raw Food Path
Network Directory
Grammer Publishing
P.O. Box 2333
New York, NY 10009-8919
(212) 353-2127

Self-Responsive Wellness Cooperative
8033 Sunset Boulevard #485
West Hollywood, CA 90046
(213) 650-4933

National Directory of Doctors Practicing Natural Hygiene

If -- in your seeking to get well and stay well without the medicine men -- you find yourself in need of advice or supervision from an Hygienic doctor, please do refer to the following list of professionals who are dedicated to offering ethical service and high standards in Hygienic care.

Charisse Basquin, D.C.
2900 St. Paul Drive, #219
Santa Rosa, CA 95405

Dr. Stanley Bass
3119 Coney Island Avenue
Brooklyn, NY 11235
Phone: (718) 648-1500

Gerald Benesh, D.C.
2050 Rockhoff Road
Escondido, CA 92026
Phone: (619) 747-4193

John Brosious, B.S., D.C.
18209 Gulf Boulevard
Redington Shores, FL 33708
Phone: (813) 392-8326

Paul W. Carlin II, D.C.
711 Bay Area Boulevard, #130
Webster, TX 77598
Phone: (713) 332-1111

Ralph C. Cinque, D.C.
Hygeia Health Retreat
439 East Main
Yorktown, TX 78164
Phone: (512) 564-3670

Dr. Christopher Deatherage, D.C., N.C.
Star Route, Box 87A
Chamois, MO 65024
Phone: (314) 943-2282

Jacques Dezavelle, D.C.
1118 Second Street
Encinitas, CA 92024
Phone: (619) 436-5151

Kenneth L. Eckhardt, D.C.
181 Lynch Creek Way, Suite 102
Petaluma, CA 94954-2313
(707) 762-1895

William Esser, N.D., D.C.
Esser's Health Ranch
P.O. Box 6629
Lake Worth, FL 33466
Phone: (407) 965-4360

Stephen Forrest, D.C.
430 Monterey Avenue, #2
Los Gatos, CA 95030
Phone: (408) 358-2188

Joel Fuhrman, M.D.
Family Health Center
427 S. Broadway
Yonkers, NY 10701
Phone: (914) 332-4090

Alan Goldhamer, D.C.
Jennifer Marano, D.C.
Kenneth Eckhardt, D.C.
Center for Chiropractic & Conservative Therapy
4310 Lichau Road
Penngrove, CA 94951
Phone: (707) 792-2325

Doug Graham, D.C.
Club Hygiene
105 Bruce Court
Marathon, FL 33050
Phone: (305) 743-3168

Thomas K. Hand, D.C.
3676 Richmond Avenue
Staten Island, NY 10312
Phone: (718) 984-5869

William Harris, M.D.
1765 Ala Moana #1880
Honolulu, HI 96815

Alan Immerman, D.C.
8229 North 53rd Street
Paradise Valley, AZ 85253
(602) 991-7131

Paul Levy, D.C.
6144 W. Roosevelt Road, 2nd Floor
Oak Park, IL 60304
Phone: (312) 865-2533

Steve Nelson, D.C.
7761 Ulmerton Road
Largo, FL 33541
Phone: (813) 535-7754

Anthony J. Penepent, M.D.
2-12 W. Park Avenue
P.O.B. 886, Long Beach, NY 11561
Phone: (516) 486-6469

David L. Reichel, D.C.
330 West Main
Perham, MN 56573
Phone: (218) 346-2330

Dr. Joel Robbins, D.C.
Health and Wellness Center
6218 South Lewis, Suite #103
Tulsa, OK 74136
Phone: (918) 742-2194

Philip C. Royal, N.C., D.C.
2607 De La Vina Street
Santa Barbara, CA 93105
Phone: (805) 569-1702

Frank Sabatino, D.C., Ph.D.
Regency Health Resort and Spa
2000 S. Ocean Drive
Hallandale, FL 33009
Phone: (305) 454-2220

Leslie H. Salov, M.D.
The Vision and Health Center
Route 4, Box 186
Whitewater, WI 53190
Phone: (414) 473-7361

D.J. Scott, D.C.
Scott's Natural Health Institute
P.O. Box 361095
Strongsville, OH 44136
Phone: (216) 671-5023

Dr. Vivian Virginia Vetrano
P.O.B. 190, Barksdale, TX 78828
Phone: (512) 234-3499

Andrew Vitko, D.C.
17023 Lorain Avenue
Cleveland, OH 44111
Phone: (216) 671-5023

Dr. Weiss, D.C.
409 E. Front Street
Bloomington, IL 61701
Phone: (309) 452-3921

Timothy R. Whelan, M.A., D.C.
Thomaston Chiropractic Center
108 Watertown Road
Thomaston, CT 06787
(203) 283-5171

Natural Hygiene Retreats

Abunda Life Health Hotel & Clinic
208 Third Avenue
Asbury Park, NY 07712

Ann Wigmore Foundation:
196 Commonwealth Avenue
Boston, MA 02116
(617) 266-6955
or
2417 West Lincoln Avenue
Montebello, CA 90640
(213) 723-1994

Club Hygiene
105 Bruce Court
Marathon, FL 33050
(305) 743-3168

Creative Health Institute
918 Union City Road
Union City, MI 49094
(517) 278-6260

Health Oasis
Route 2, P.O. Box 10
Tilly, AR 72679
(501) 496-2364

Helen Lamar
P.O. Box 1482
Santa Cruz, CA 95060
(408) 426-8546

Hippocrates Health Institute
1443 Palmdale Court
West Palmdale, FL 33441
(407) 471-8876

Hygeia Health Retreat
439 East Main Street
Yorktown, TX 78164
(512) 564-3670

Optimum Health Institute of San Diego
(formerly Hippocrates West)
6970 Central Avenue
Lemon Grove, CA 92045
(619) 464-3346

Pawling Health Manor
P.O. Box 401
Hyde Park, NY 12538
(914) 889-4141

Scott's Natural Health Institute
P.O. Box 361095
Strongsville, Ohio 44136
(216) 238-6930

Juice Bars and Restaurants

Beverly Hills Juice Club
8382 Beverly Boulevard
Los Angeles, California
(213) 655-8300

Cafe La De Da
2010 Jimmy Durante Blvd.
Del Mar, California
(619) 792-2221
(Open for lunch and dinner only. Call for hours.)

Fountain of Juice
1163 First Street
Encinitas, California
(619) 944-0612

Garden Taste
1555 Camino Del Mar
(in the Del Mar Plaza)
Del Mar, California
(619) 793-1500

Get Juiced
1423 Fifth Street
Santa Monica, California
(213) 395-8177

Govinda's Natural
Foods Restaurant
3102 University Avenue
San Diego, California
(619) 284-4826

I Love Juicy
(3 locations:)

7174 Melrose Avenue
Los Angeles, California
(213) 935-7247
&
10845 Lindbrook Drive
Westwood, California
(310) 208-3242
&
Hampton Drive
Venice, California
(310) 399-1318

Ki's Juice Bar (I)
206 Birmingham Drive
Cardiff by the Sea, California
(619) 436-5236

Ki's Juice Bar (II)
(no relation to Ki's I)
407 C Street (between 4th and 5th Avenues)
San Diego, California
(619) 232-8208

La Hood's Natural Juices
Grand Central Market
317 S. Broadway
Los Angeles, California
(213) 629-2787

The Vegetarian
431 West 13th Avenue
Escondido, California
(619) 740-9596

Vegetarian Groups

Jewish Vegetarian Society
P.O. Box 5722
Baltimore, MD 21208
(301) 486-4948

Live Food Singles Club -- World Wide
11015 Cumpston Street
North Hollywood, CA 91601
(818) 763-1000

North American Vegetarianism Society
P.O. Box 72
Dolgeville, NY 13329

San Francisco Vegetarian Society, Inc.
1450 Broadway, No. 4
San Francisco, CA 94109
(415) 775-6874

Vegetarian Information Service, Inc.
P.O. Box 5888
Bethesda, MD 20814
(301) 530-1737

Vegetarian Society, Inc.
P.O. Box 34427
Los Angeles, CA 90034
(213) 281-1907

Special Mention

The Essene Gospel of Peace
(about Jesus and fasting; $2.50 total cost)
IBS International
P.O. Box 205
Matsqui, BC VOX 1SO
Canada

or from

The Gerston Institute
P.O. Box 430
Bonita, CA 91908

Other Resources

Bodhi Tree Bookstore
8585 Melrose Avenue
West Hollywood, CA 90069
(310) 659-1733

Paras Dea, Reflexologist
5666 La Jolla Boulevard, Suite 174
La Jolla, CA 92037
(619) 621-9047
Pager: (619) 260-9463

International Institute of Reflexology
P.O. Box 12642
St. Petersburg, FL 33733-2642
(818) 343-4811

Dr. Vivian V. Vetrano
Box 190
Barksdale, TX 78828-0190
(210) 234-3499
Write for information about Dr. Vetrano's videos, tapes, newsletter, health retreat, and Health Information Services (telephone counseling).

Dr. William F. Welles
6565 Balboa Avenue, Suite A
San Diego, CA 92111
(619) 541-1440

GLOSSARY

Acid: A typically sour, water-soluble compound capable of reacting with a base to form a salt.

Alkaline: Having the properties of an alkali; having a pH over 7.

Alkalosis: A pathological condition resulting from accumulation of base minerals or excessive loss of acid minerals from the body; a condition of increased alkalinity of the blood and tissues.

Amino Acid: A building block in the construction of proteins. All proteins are composed of one or more of the 23 amino acids.

Carbohydrates: A group of closely related organic compounds containing carbon, hydrogen, and oxygen. They are used in the maintenance of the functional activity of cells, and they serve as structural and reserve cell material for plants. Carbohydrates are formed in plants in the process of photosynthesis. Along with proteins and fats, they comprise the major components of living matter (both plant and animal).

Digestion: The process by which the complex materials of food are broken down into simpler substances in preparation for their entrance into the bloodstream.

Enzyme: A protein that acts as a catalyst to reduce complex substances to simple and more usable components.

Fermentation: Decomposition (as opposed to digestion) of sugar and starch (carbohydrates), and their conversion by microorganisms (bacteria) to carbon dioxide, alcohol, acetic acid, and lactic acid.

Gastric: Pertaining to the stomach.

Health: A condition in which all functions of the body and mind are normally active. A state of complete physical, mental, or social well-being and not merely the absence of disease or infirmity. Wholeness.

Hygiene: The science of health. The word is derived from Hygeia, the Greek goddess of health.

Hygienist: Meaning natural hygienist, one who practices natural hygiene.

Inorganic: As applied to minerals, a mineral that exists in the soil, air, or water that has not been absorbed or elaborated by plants.

Insalivation: The process by which saliva is secreted to help moisten food and to initiate digestion.

Metabolism: The building-up and breaking-down processes of the body as a whole.

Nerve energy: Generated under the condition of sleep, nerve energy is created by the brain and nervous system. Toxemia greatly affects the level of nerve energy.

Nutrition: The sum total of all the processes that interact to supply our nutritive needs.

Omnivore: An animal that is physiologically and anatomically adapted to feeding on both plant life and animal life.

Pathogenic: That which is toxic or obnoxious within the organism; that which causes the body to react with an infection or disease. Pathogenic means, literally, disease-generating.

pH factor: A measure of acidity, neutrality, or alkalinity of a liquid or a solid.

Protein: The primary substance of life; the building material of organisms. Composed of amino acids in an endless variety of linkages.

Putrefaction: Decomposition of proteins and their conversion by microorganisms to poisonous substances.

Toxemia: A condition arising from toxins in the blood in excess of the norm of that formed by regular catabolic and metabolic processes.

Unsaturated fats: The existence of open-linked fatty acid chains which have the capability to combine with other nutrients.

Preface to Catalog Sheets

By selling the products and books on the next pages, I do not wish to give the appearance of commercialism to this book and therefore distract from its message. If you follow the instructions in this book, that will be sufficient to stop your indigestion. The products are simply an adjunct to the program. The books are to enhance your knowledge about natural hygiene.

CATALOG SHEETS
Catalog Sheet -- Source #1

The Welles Wedge™

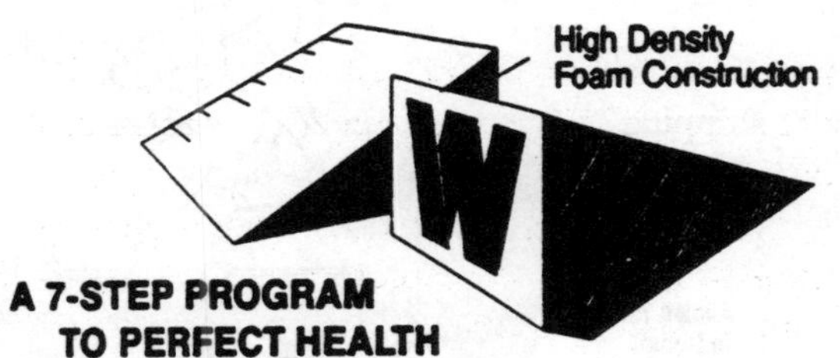

The Need

The need for the wedges began when man adopted two faulty cultural habits
1. Elevated heels in shoes
2. Use of the raised Western Toilet instead of squatting

These two faulty cultural habits have left our calf, hamstring and pelvic muscles shortened and imbalanced.
This leaves great room for improvement in all aspects of human performance.
The use of the Welles Wedges restores structural balance and health which is our heritage.

MANUFACTURED BY:

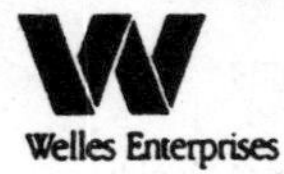

Welles Enterprises

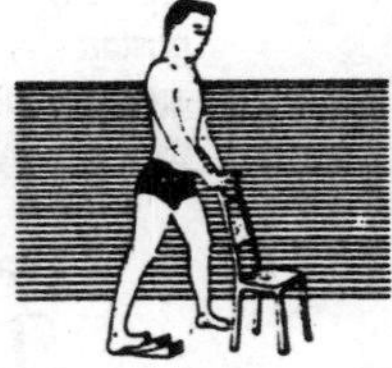

Isolation and stretching of the calf muscles and the hamstrings are made easy with the Welles Wedges. Angle of stretch varied by overlapping the two wedges.

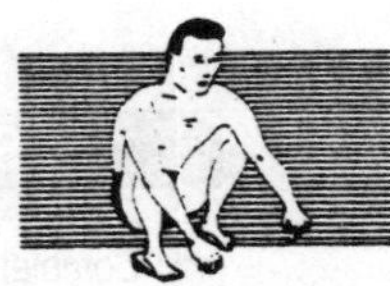

Three wonderful squatting postures which have a dramatic effect on your low back geometry are accomplished with the Welles Wedges.

The Benefit

(in minutes daily)

- Dramatically improved energy levels
- Reduction of low back and hip pain
- Improves dropped arches and ankle problems
- Improved athletic performance and reduced injuries
- Re-newed sexual energy
- Eases childbirth
- Remarkably improves bowel function
- Flattens the abdomen
- Improves Posture

Wedges come with complete instructions for 4 calf and hamstring stretches and 3 squatting exercises.

Only **$8.95** a pair
(plus $1.75 shipping)

Order form on last page.

Catalog Sheet -- Source #1
(continued)

The Welles Step

PATENT PENDING

$59
plus $5.90 shipping

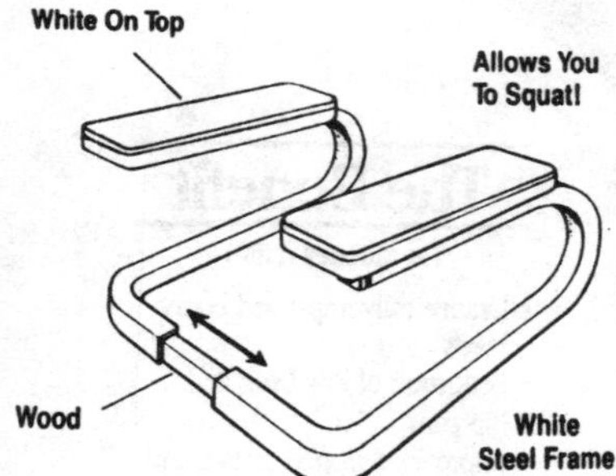

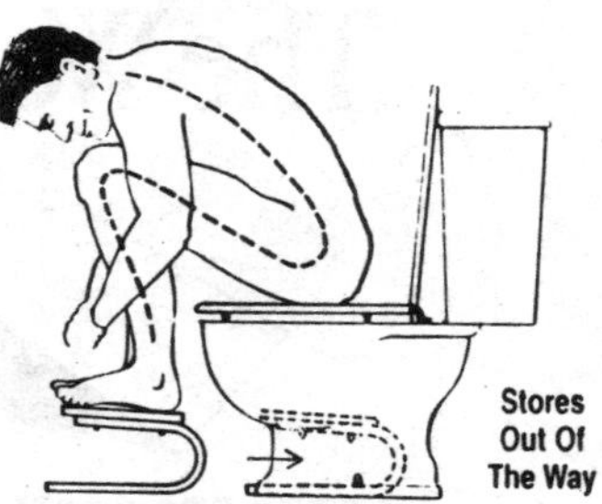

People were intended to squat. They squatted throughout history. With this posture the abdominal wall and bowel are supported as we bear down. This is nature's way.

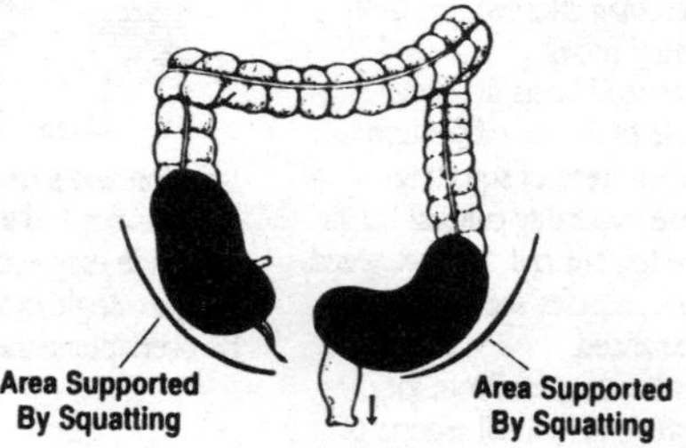

FEATURES

Fully recesses under toilet when not in use

Adjustable width to fit your toilet

Angled steps gently stretch calves and allow you to vary height of feet

White powder-coated frame and top quality, non-skid step top assures many years of healthful use.

POSITIVE BENEFITS

- ✚ Complete Bowel Evacuation
- ✚ Freedom from Laxatives
- ✚ Fewer Hemorrhoids & Hernias
- ✚ Fewer Varicose Veins
- ✚ A Clean Bloodstream - Vibrant Health

Order form on last page.

Catalog Sheet -- Source #1
(continued)

The Welles Arch™

PATENT PENDING

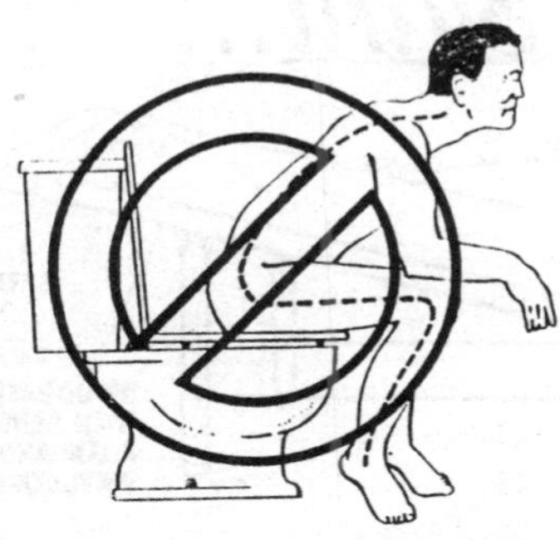

$39
plus $3.90 shipping

Reflex Point Massage Rollers

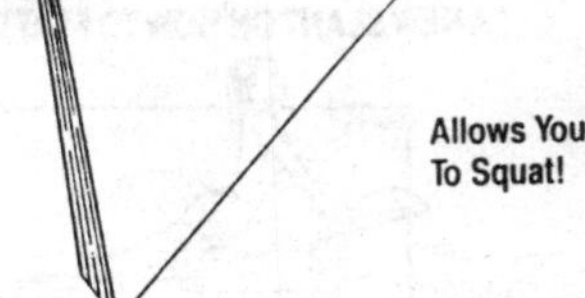

Allows You To Squat!

The Modern Toilet was a great mistake. It leaves these two areas of the abdominal wall and bowel unsupported as we bear down. (See red area on illustration below).

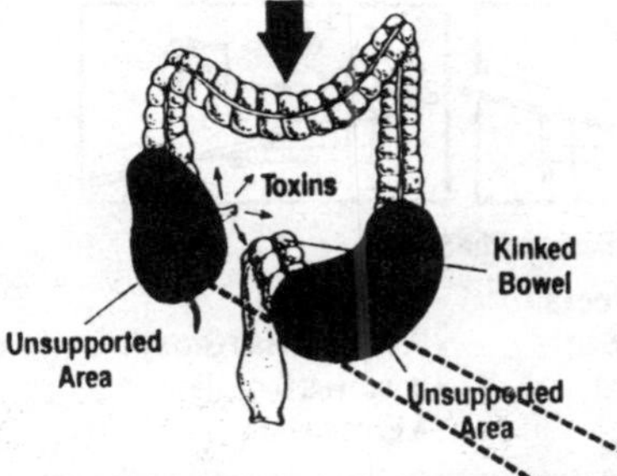

FEATURES

Reflex Rollers stimulate the bowel reflex on the foot.

Tender Reflex Areas

Check These Reflexes On You

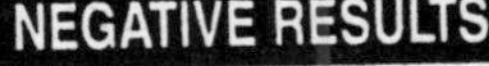

NEGATIVE RESULTS

- ⊘ Incomplete Elimination of These Areas
- ⊘ A Kinked Bowel - Fecal Stagnation
- ⊘ Toxins enter into The Bloodstream
- ⊘ Hemorrhoids - Varicose Veins
- ⊘ A Diseased Colon and Body

Order form on last page.

Catalog Sheet -- Source #1
(continued)

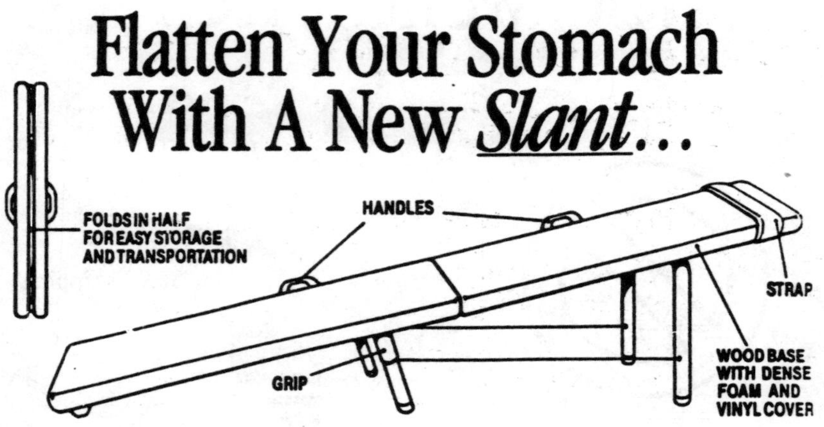

THE WELLES *SLANT*™

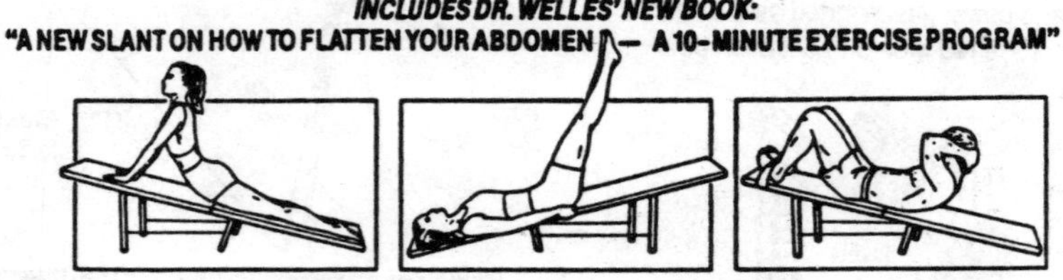

Benefits of Lying and Exercising on the Slant:

- Flattens Your Abdomen
- Clears Complexion
- Natural Face Lift
- Tones Your Buttocks
- Reduces Body Sag
- More Sex Appeal
- Weight Loss
- Promotes Hair Growth
- Improves Digestion & Elimination

$149 plus $15 shipping. Book included:
Flatten Your Stomach with a New Slant

Order form on last page.

Send SASE for reviews of books of interest. To order, circle the number and price of each book you want.

1. *The Great AIDS Hoax*,
   T.C. Fry, 320 pp $13.00
2. *Toxemia Explained/True Healing Art*,
   Dr. J.H. Tilden, 128 pp $8.00
3. *I Live on Fruit*,
   T.C. Fry and Essi Honiball, 112 pp $8.00
4. *Overcoming Asthma*,
   Beth Snodgrass, 64 pp $4.00
5. *Vaccinations Do Not Protect*,
   E. McBean, Ph.D., N.D., 48 pp $3.00
6. *The Cruel Hoax Called Herpes Genitalis*,
   Fry/Shelton, 96 pp. $8.00
7. *Superior Nutrition**,
   Dr. Herbert Shelton, 128 pp $8.00
8. *The Myth of Medicine*,
   T.C. Fry, 64 pp $4.00
9. *Fasting: The Fastest Way to Vibrant Health*,
   T.C. Fry, 64 pp $4.00
10. VEGGIE DELIGHT Dehydrated
    Vegetable Seasoning, 8 oz $10.00

To order: Include $2.00 shipping for orders under $15.00, 25¢ for each additional book. When ordering Veggie Delight with a book order, add $1.00 shipping. Order on last page.

---

*A most important classic book.

Send SASE for reviews of books of interest. To order, circle the number and price of each book you want.

1. *How to Break a Bad Habit*, Dr. Ralph Cinque $10.00
2. *Slanting: A Complete Guide for the Body, Mind, & Spirit*, Sharlin Leslie $13.00
3. *Problems with Meat*, John Scharffenberg $6.00
4. *Diets Don't Work*, Bob Schwartz $11.00
5. *The Salt Conspiracy*, Victoria BidWell $6.00
6. *Self Care vs. Medical Care*†, Hannah Allen $3.00
7. *Medical Drugs on Trial -- Verdict Guilty!*†, Dr. Keki Sidhwa $4.00
8. *Fasting Can Save Your Life*, Dr. Herbert Shelton $8.00
9. *Why Christians Get Sick*, by the Rev. George H. Malkmus $7.95
10. Veggie Volt (Dehydrated Vegetable Seasoning), 16 oz $16.00*
11. Hot Water Bottle -- Super King Size (18" x 24") $22.00*

*Postage included. †Highly recommended.

Add $2.00 for the first book ordered and 25¢ for each additional book. Order form on last page.

Catalog Sheet -- Source #4

THE GARDEN OF EDEN RAW FRUIT & VEGETABLE RECIPES

By Phyllis Avery

(all vegan—no milk products)

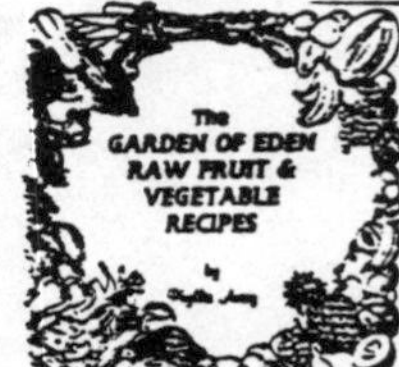

<u>FRUIT RECIPES:</u> HORS D'OEUVRES, FRUIT DISHES, FRUIT SYRUPS, FRUIT SHAKES and FRUIT DRINKS!

<u>VEGETABLE RECIPES:</u> HORS D'OEUVRES, SOUPS, DIPS, DRESSINGS (made without vinegar, mayonnaise, or oil), and 50 MAIN DISHES.

Plus an introduction to natural hygiene, a two-page food combining chart and basic food-combining principles, a chapter on selecting and storing fruits and vegetables, and a list of natural hygiene organizations.

The recipes conform to the principles of natural hygiene.

126 Pages $10.95

THE 10-MINUTE VEGETARIAN COOKBOOK

By Phyllis Avery

True Transition Recipes

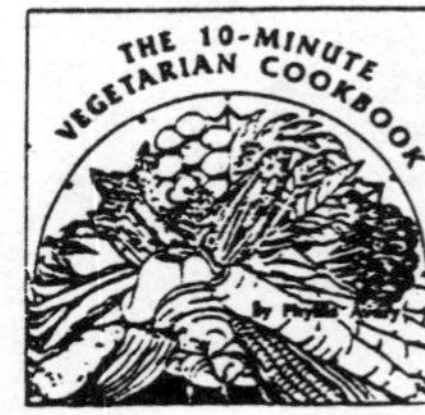

Quick, nutritious dishes that are steamed from 4 to 10 minutes. The main ingredient in all recipes are fresh vegetables. All recipes are entrees. The soups and salads are hearty enough for a complete meal. No-nonsense recipes — all ingredients are common items, with minimal use of processed foods.

The 143-page book offers 192 recipes. $10.95

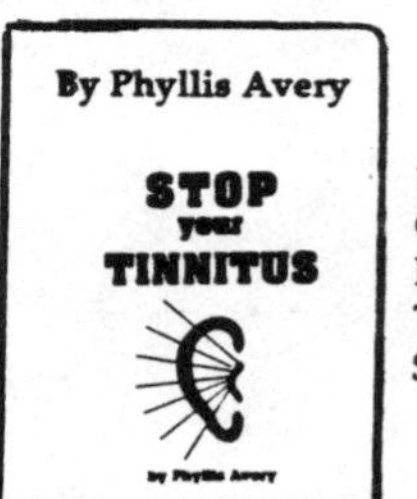

STOP YOUR TINNITUS:

Causes, Preventatives, Treatments

184 page book offers: External Causative Agents, Chemicals, Internal Causative Disorders, Physiological Intervention, Psychological Intervention, Alimentary Intervention, Telephone Hearing Screening Test, 13 pages of Glossary terms, 16 pages of Resources, 108 Medical and Scientific References.

$14.95

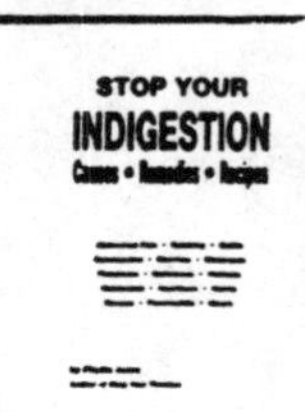

STOP YOUR INDIGESTION

Causes, Remedies, Recipes

This three-part, 240-page book explains 16 reasons why people suffer from indigestion. The second section offers remedies for particular diseases that develop from indigestion. The third section has recipes that prevent indigestion. The book also has a resources list and a glossary.

$14.95

Add $1.75 shipping for 1 book, 25¢ for each additional book. When shipped to California, add 7% sales tax. See next page for order form.

Order Form

Total from Source #1 __________

Total from Source #2 __________

Total from Source #3 __________

Total from Source #4 __________

Grand Total __________

Send to:
Hygeia Publishing Company
1358 Fern Place
Vista, CA 92083

Name ....

Street ....

City/State/Zip ....

....

Order Form

Total from Source #1 ____________

Total from Source #2 ____________

Total from Source #3 ____________

Total from Source #4 ____________

Grand Total ____________

Send to:
Hygeia Publishing Company
1358 Fern Place
Vista, CA 92083

Name . . . .

Street . . . .

City/State/Zip . . . .

. . . .